The Ethics of Sp[ ]

The book aims to establish a criti[ ] [ ]
across the range of sporting disci[ ]. It will address questions such as:

Are the increasingly intrusive[ ] [ ] Georgia Law requires Library materials to
to autonomy and privacy [ ] [s] be returned or replacement costs paid.
Failure to comply with this law is a
Could there be a moral oblig[ ] [ju] misdemeanor. (O.C.G.A. 20-5-53)
and

How should the goals of sp[c] [ ]ewed from the perspective of rationing
scarce health care resources?

This book was published as a special issue in *Sport, Ethics and Philosophy*.

Claudio M. Tamburrini is a senior researcher at the Stockholm Bioethics Centre in the Department of Philosophy, Stockholm University, Sweden.

Torbjörn Tännsjö is a Professor of Practical Philosophy at Stockholm University, Sweden.

Ethics and Sport

Series editors
Mike McNamee
University of Wales Swansea
Jim Parry
University of Leeds
Heather Reid
Morningside College

The Ethics and Sport series aims to encourage critical reflection on the practice of sport, and to stimulate professional evaluation and development. Each volume explores new work relating to philosophical ethics and the social and cultural study of ethical issues. Each is different in scope, appeal, focus and treatment but a balance is sought between local and international focus, perennial and contemporary issues, level of audience, teaching and research application, and variety of practical concerns.

Also available in this series:

The Ethics of Sports Medicine

Edited by Claudio Tamburrini and Torbjörn Tännsjö

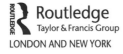

Routledge
Taylor & Francis Group

LONDON AND NEW YORK

First published 2009 by Routledge
2 Park Square, Milton Park, Abingdon, Oxon, OX14 4RN

Simultaneously published in the USA and Canada
by Routledge
711 Third Avenue, New York, NY 10017

Routledge is an imprint of the Taylor & Francis Group, an informa business

© 2009 Taylor & Francis

First issued in paperback 2013

Typeset in Myriad by KGL Ltd., Southampton, UK

British Library Cataloguing in Publication Data
A catalogue record for this book is available from the British Library

ISBN13: 978-0-415-85367-5 (pbk)
ISBN13: 978-0-415-48051-2 (hbk)

Contents

Introduction

TRANSCENDING HUMAN LIMITATIONS

Claudio M. Tamburrini and Torbjörn Tännsjö

In the wake of the explosion of commercialised professional sports, sport medicine has evolved as an increasingly independent area within the general medical landscape. This phenomenon however has not been accompanied by a parallel development in sport medical ethics. Yet, what precisely are the aims pursued within sport medicine? Its scientific ethos might be summarised by the goal of *transcending limitations*. Unlike general medical practice, which only recently incorporated among its goals and pursuits the amelioration of non-pathological conditions, sport medicine has from its very beginning been driven by the ambition of helping humans of a certain kind – more precisely, professional elite athletes – to surpass the limits of what hitherto has been considered as possible for the species to achieve in a sport arena.

This development poses new questions regarding the special circumstances under which medical work is conducted in sports as well as about the central ethical notions that characterise sport medicine. Apparently some of the central ethical concepts usually applied in general medical practice are given a different content when applied in sport medical contexts. While core moral notions such as privacy and autonomy are underlined in the current medical ethical debate, these notions acquire a rather different resonance when applied to sport medicine ethics. In general medicine, patients are seen as autonomous agents, granted the right to decide for themselves whether to submit to a particular treatment or not. Not to undergo treatment, or interrupting it once it has been started, might be related to risks for the patient's health. Her right to decide for herself is nonetheless respected. In sport medicine ethics, however, a more paternalistic approach seems to be preponderant. Athletes are not allowed to submit themselves to training methods or techniques that are judged, either by the sport community or by sport officials or both, as too risky. An athlete's consent to undergoing a certain training technique seems to be of less weight than a patient's consent to submitting herself to a still unsafe treatment. Moreover, even some safe medical measures, intended to enhance the performance of the athlete, are often prohibited in the sport context, now with reference to the ethos of sport rather than with reference to health hazards. While for instance the concert violinist may use beta blockers in order to enhance his or her performance, this cure is proscribed in the world of sports.

Nevertheless, parallel to this trend of risk aversion, a certain predisposition to accept more risks is obviously prevalent in the world of sports. Which attitude should sport doctors adopt faced with this fact? This issue is addressed in the first chapter of this volume. In 'Doctoring risk: Responding to risk-taking in athletes', Linley Anderson addresses the question of athletes who wish to compete in spite of a high risk of injury.

Overriding their choices could be considered to be unnecessarily overbearing or paternalistic. However, Anderson believes that simply accepting all risk-taking as the voluntary choice of an individual fails to acknowledge the context of high-level sport and the circumstances in which an athlete may be being coerced or in some other way making a less than voluntary choice. In this article, the author explores the ways a sports doctor might respond in order to ensure that the athlete's choice is indeed voluntary, and characterises the circumstances under which limits might be placed in an attempt to balance the athlete's aims against some set of ideals of good health or medical ends.

Not only with respect to risk, a trend towards liberalisation is visible. This is true also with respect to some drugs and training methods that were earlier seen to be at variance with the ethos of sport. And the two themes, the one related to health and the other to the ethos of sports, are in close connection with each other. A traditional argument advanced by those who oppose the prohibition on doping says that with no doping ban it would be possible to have safer doping under medical control. Starting from a distinction between self-employed sportspersons and sportspersons who get their main income from an employer, Soren Holm develops in his article 'Doping under medical control – conceptually possible but impossible in the world of professional sports?' a game-theoretical argument to show that this positive scenario would probably not occur. As some sport doctors seem to act as agents of their employers rather than on behalf of their patients/sportspersons, we should not expect them to give impartial advice to their patients in conditions when they are contracted by an employer. Similarly, if sportspersons are employed by a club or a national team, it is also highly unlikely that they would be given the choice between doping or not doping by their employers. If we instead focus on sportspersons who are self-employed, and assuming they will strive to maximise their competitive advantages, we should not expect either that they will refrain from testing new, still unsafe substances if the doping ban were lifted. Therefore, Holm concludes, even without the ban it seems unrealistic to expect a safer working situation for professional athletes regarding doping.

On a more general level, it might be argued that failing to situate doping issues within the current scientific and ethical discussion on enhancement risks creating a professional area, elite sports, with mandatory principles and regulations that are divorced from what is usually accepted in outside society. In his article 'Genetics, bioethics and sport', Andy Miah discloses what he sees as methodological limitations of anti-doping due to its reluctance to address the doping issue within a broader bioethical debate about genetics, the ethics of enhancement and the use of medicine in sport more generally. In his view, the kind of arguments being raised during the last decades in bioethical discussions have not yet informed the doping debate to an appropriate degree. In a world that permits the use of gene transfer technology for therapeutic purposes, how could sports authorities prohibit genetically modified athletes to compete, just because they were genetically modified? Nor have fundamental issues regarding the legitimacy of anti-doping work been properly addressed either. For one thing, Miah argues, the global context of sport raises challenging philosophical issues about the universality of moral principles. Are sport ethics universal? Immersed in a reality that remains befuddled by the human cloning debate and the internationality of ethics related to human genetics, the World Anti-Doping Agency (WADA) is bypassing that confusion and asserting what is right and proper for humans by prohibiting gene doping on the basis of a contested assumption that there are unified codes of ethics in sport. Once we adopt a proper approach to (gene) doping as one among the various techniques for human enhancement, Miah concludes, we might find that a straightforward mapping of medical ethics onto sport ethics is not justified.

Also regarding the issue of privacy there appears to be a divergence between traditional medical ethical codes and the kind of ethical code that might be formulated for the sport medicine profession. Often, individuals have the right not to disclose information about their genetic constitution, for instance when signing a policy with a private insurance company. The protection of privacy is central in the health-care system as well as in other areas of society. This, however, does not seem to be the case in the world of professional, elite sports. At present, WADA is funding research projects aimed at developing testing methods to discover so called 'gene doping'. Apparently athletes do not enjoy a similar protection against disclosing their genetic constitution as common people and other professional groups.

Sportspersons' privacy is the issue raised in by Sarah Teetzel. Probably few people would argue that the issue of athlete's privacy is an all-or-nothing matter. Thus, a proper question to pose is what degree of privacy athletes can expect and demand in the era of genetic technology in sport. In her article 'Respecting privacy in detecting illegitimate enhancements in athletes', she claims that 'Both the method of conducting random unannounced testing and the requirement that athletes supply their whereabouts at all times, so that anti-doping agencies will be able to locate them in order to conduct doping tests, are indicative of the lack of concern given to athletes' privacy'. Accordingly, using tests to detect genetic enhancements in sport, and consequently doping violations, is problematic because testing requires access to athletes' genetic information. A usual answer to these queries from official sporting bodies has been to stress the fact that athletes after all voluntarily agree to submit themselves to the testing procedures. Teetzel questions that argument, underlining the fact that athletes cannot refuse to take a doping test without risking severe sanctions. This fact renders the supposed voluntariness of their consent in her view suspect and morally problematic.

One of the most discussed questions in relation to the utilisation of enhancement techniques in sports is the issue of autonomy. Can new technologies (included so-called gene doping) be expected to increase athletes' autonomy (no limits on their choice of training methods is imposed upon them), or will they instead create a situation in which most of them will be compelled to dope in order not to loose competitive advantages? In 'Genetic enhancement, sports and relational autonomy', Susan Sherwin asks which attitude we should take towards the development of the new technology. Should we welcome such innovations, should we resign ourselves to their inevitable appearance or should we instead actively resist their development and widespread adoption? In her contribution to this issue, Sherwin proposes we start considering this question not as a matter of individual choice but rather as a question of social policy. According to the free choice argument, we should allow individual users to decide if they wish to accept the risks involved in genetic modification, provided that they have available full and accurate information about the risks and benefits involved. In response to this argument, Sherwin pleads for replacing traditional interpretations of autonomy with a relational alternative that conceives of persons as (at least partially) constituted by social interactions. As relational theorists deny that people discover their own values by introspection and believe that values are formed through social engagement, she asks us not to focus on the question 'what does a person want to do now?', but rather on 'what are the processes by which he has come to hold his current preferences?' Hence, Sherwin concludes, 'autonomy requires more than an ability to make a rational informed choice – it also requires a social context that does not encourage selection of options that are contrary to an agent's overall well-being (and are within the realm of society's ability to support).'

Another aspect in which general medical practice and sport medicine seem to differ is regarding the conception of the body. In medicine, the human body is mainly seen as a natural entity to be cured if affected by disease, but not as a proper object of engineering and instrumental use. Sport medicine, instead, seems more prone to adopt this latter approach. An interesting question is whether the view still dominating in medical practice in general will be eroded by sport medicine practice. Or has it already been eroded, as it is suggested by the various medical specialisations devoted to enhancing the human body (plastic surgery, incipient genetic technology to improve people's heath, the use of medicines to enhance life quality and so on)? At a deeper level is the question of how to relate to the limitations of our human condition. Should we accept them as constitutive elements of our human nature, however defined? Or should we instead see these limitations as merely contingent fact imposed upon us by our natural evolution and, therefore, as proper objects to be modified through scientific endeavours? This issue is addressed by Mike McNamee in a controversial article 'Transhumanism, technology and the moral topography of sports medicine', where he challenges the assumptions of transhumanism, an ideology that seeks to complete the merely 'half-baked' project of human nature. Pointing out to the common ground the enhancement ideology shares with elite sports, Mc Namee objects to what he sees as the morally repugnant transformation of a noble practice and tries to set up the moral limits of sports medicine. His article includes the reminder: 'We are mortal beings. Our vulnerability to disease and death, far from something we can overcome or eliminate, represents natural limits both for morality and medicine generally and sports medicine in particular.'

A recently advanced objection to the possibility of criticising enhancement technologies on the grounds of their supposed dehumanising character states that we do not have an agreed-upon notion of what it is to be human. In his contribution, Leon Culbertson rejects the idea that a moral evaluation of performance enhancement technologies requires a clear idea of humanness. In his view, it is the negative form 'dehumanise' rather than the affirmative form 'humanness' that is dominant. Following Wittgenstein, the author claims that 'dehumanise' is one of those words whose meaning follows from its use. Thus we can understand concrete cases of dehumanising activities either from the context or the contrast that is drawn in each particular case. Culbertson's conclusion is that the philosophy of sport should abandon the idea that moral evaluation of performance enhancement should rest on grasping the essence of the term 'human' and only can be validated by an adequate conception of humanness.

Scientific and technological progress within genetics has also raised fundamental questions regarding traditional notions of justice that have been challenged in new ways in the world of professional elite sports. For example, could there be a moral obligation to correct injustices produced by the genetic lottery, i.e. in people's natural endowments? If so, does it follow from that obligation that sport medicine should engage in equalising the conditions of competition between athletes rather than engaging in finding methods to disclose 'gene cheaters'? Should society compensate for congenital, 'natural', differences between people? And would it then be appropriate that sport organisations compensate for 'natural' differences between athletes, for instance by creating new categories in competition, thus separating the best from the worst genetically endowed athletes? All these issues raise particular worries for the broadly embraced ideal of fairness in competition, one of the central tenets of the ethos of sports according to many authors. In his contribution, Christian Lenk sets out to show that enhancement activities are contradictory to basic requirements and preconditions of sports competitions, mainly a basic equality of opportunities for all competitors as well as a clear causal connection – which he calls 'authorship' – between a specific performance and an individual athlete. In his article 'Is enhancement in sport really unfair? Arguments on the concept of competition and equality of opportunities', he claims that the situation in which one party in sports competitions has a decisive advantage not because of training and performance but because of enhancement technologies, is unfair and should therefore be ruled out. To avoid that effect in a context in which doping were allowed, it would then be necessary to create an institution to guarantee the same level of performance enhancement for all teams. Obviously, Lenk concludes, this seems to be a worse scenario than the present state of regulation in which the doping ban is upheld.

Following up the discussion on the probable effects of new genetic technologies on sports and society, Claudio Tamburrini – one of the editors of this volume – focuses on the question of distributive justice. He pictures a future scenario in which most of the new therapeutic and enhancement techniques will probably be quite expensive, with the consequence that their use is practically monopolised by the rich, to the detriment of all those who are not in a position to afford genetic treatments. This notwithstanding, Tamburrini argues that the health-care inequality that probably will follow from the adoption of genetic technology is hardly a reason to reject the new technology, as in that case we would have to reject any new medicine or medical technique that cannot be made available to all people at once. Perhaps the poor of the present will not have access to the new technologies. But the have-nots of the future certainly will do, when the new techniques are made available to everyone, as we have already witnessed in the past regarding for instance antibiotics. Thus, Tamburrini concludes, the enhanced new world that would follow the introduction of genetic technology poses no serious threat either to elite sports or to society and should therefore be welcome.

A particular instantiation of 'the genetic lottery argument' regards what measures would be appropriate to take in order to reduce differences in performances between the sexes (what is usually referred to as 'the muscle gap'). Adding new fuel to a debate that took off in our previous anthology,[1] Kutte Jönsson charges our proposal on 'Bio-Amazons' with not being radical enough. In the closing contribution to this issue, 'Who's afraid of Stella Walsh? On gender, "gene cheaters" and the promises of cyborg athletes', he argues that 'Although their [Tamburrini and Tännsjö's] argument works in favour of the idea of individuals crossing sex/gender barriers, it still entails the acceptance of the concept of gender, and the concept of gender differentiates bodies into certain (gender) norms, and that involves and promotes (gender) discrimination.' Jönsson's view is that only in a world of asexual cyborgs can gender discrimination – both in sport and in society – be successfully neutralised. Rather than trying to abolish sex and gender discrimination by social, cultural and political means (as our critics have argued against us) or by biological means (as we argue), Jönsson believes that we should abolish sex and gender as normative and discriminating categorisations.

All these issues raise several theoretical and practical questions, both with regard to medical ethics and the ethics of sport medicine. For instance, how should the goals of sports medicine be viewed from the perspective of rationing scarce health-care resources? Should sports medicine be restricted by rules from the sports community regarding which performance-enhancing activities are tolerated in that sector? Or should sports medicine rather direct what is to be accepted within the world of sports? Perhaps not surprisingly, during the work of compiling the material for this book, we have come to realise that the differences – rather, the divergent and competing character of many of the contributions presented in this volume – can be traced to a radically different approach to the question of whether we should accept limitations (physical, cognitive, in mood and life span) as constitutive of human nature, or whether we should instead see them as contingent, historically determined biological facts that can – and should? – be transcended by enhancements.

While we hope this collection will result in a number of theoretical and practical insights on the various issues presented above, we also see it as a further contribution to the mutually enriching interchange between sport philosophers and bio-ethicists started with the publication of our two previous sport ethical anthologies. In that regard, we wish to thank the Bank of Sweden Third Centenary Foundation for supporting the conference on human enhancement out of which most of the articles presented here originated, as well as the European Union Sixth Framework Programme – Deepening Understanding on Ethical Issues and our associate researchers within the Enhance project for their contributions to the realisation of this volume. The results of this collaboration between different European universities and scholars lie now before the reader as a starting-point for a systematic reflection on the specific character and particular challenges posed by sport medicine ethics, a still neglected area of research.

NOTES

1.   See Tamburrini and Tännsjö 2005.

REFERENCES

TAMBURRINI, C. and T. TÄNNSJÖ, eds. 2005. *Genetic Technology and Sport – Ethical Questions.* London and New York: Routledge.

DOCTORING RISK: RESPONDING TO RISK-TAKING IN ATHLETES

Lynley Anderson

Athletes who wish to compete in spite of high risk of injury can prove a challenge for sports doctors. Overriding an athlete's choices could be considered to be unnecessarily overbearing or paternalistic. However simply accepting all risk-taking as the voluntary choice of an individual fails to acknowledge the context of high-level sport and the circumstances in which an athlete may be being coerced or in some other way be making a less than voluntary choice. Restricting the voluntary choices of an athlete may still be possible but under very limited circumstances. This article explores the ways a sports doctor might respond in ensuring a choice is indeed voluntary and, if so, under what circumstances limits might be placed. Responding to such risk-taking by, for example, limiting the actions of an athlete or assisting them to compete, involves attempting to balance the athlete's aims against some set of ideals of good health or medical ends.

Resumen

Los atletas que deseen competir a pesar del alto riesgo de lesión pueden resultar ser un desafío para los médicos deportivos. Hacer caso omiso de las decisiones del atleta puede ser considerado innecesariamente prepotente o paternalista. Sin embargo el aceptar simplemente todo riesgo como la elección voluntaria de un individuo no tiene en cuenta el contexto del deporte de alta competición y las circunstancias en las que un atleta puede estar siendo coaccionado o tomando una decisión de una manera no muy voluntaria que se diga. La restricción de las decisiones personales de un atleta puede ser todavía posible pero bajo circunstancias muy limitadas. Este artículo explora las maneras en la que un médico deportivo podría responder para asegurarse de que una elección es realmente voluntaria, y de ser así, bajo que circunstancias se pordrían establecer límites. El responder a la toma de tales riesgos, por ejemplo, limitando las acciones del atleta o ayudándoles en la competición, implica el intentar equilibrar las metas del atleta con ciertos ideales sobre la salud o los objetivos médicos.

Zusammenfassung

Athleten die trotz hohen Verletzungsrisikos an Wettkämpfen teilnehmen möchten, stellen Sportmediziner vor gewisse Herausforderungen. Sich über den Willen des Sportlers hinwegzusetzen könnte als unbotmäßige Dominanz oder als Bevormundung verstanden werden. Jedoch zu glauben, die Übernahme von Risiken sei nur die Entscheidung des Individuums, ignoriert die Tatsache, dass im leistungssportlichen Umfeld Athleten evtl. gezwungen sind bzw. nicht ganz freiwillig gewisse Entscheidungen treffen. Die Einschränkung der Entscheidungsfreiheit eines Sportlers kann geboten sein, jedoch nur unter ganz bestimmten Umständen. Dieser Artikel untersucht die Handlungsmöglichkeiten der Sportmediziner zur Sicherstellung einer freien Entscheidung, sowie der möglichen Umstände zu deren Einschränkung. Reaktionen auf derartiges Risikoverhalten, wie die Einschränkung der Handlungsfreiheit eines Athleten oder aber auch die Unterstützung um Einsatzfähig zu sein, ist Verbunden mit dem Versuch die Ziele des Sportlers mit den Idealvorstellungen von Gesundheit und medizinischen Absichten in Einklang zu bringen.

摘要

對於有一些運動員想要參與一些具有高危險傷害的比賽，這對運動醫師來說是一種挑戰。 若因為這樣就去剝奪運動員的選擇權，可能會被視為一種不必要的承擔或是一種父權主義的作用。不過，若簡單接受所有危險皆因個人的自主選擇，則會失去了解到高水準運動比賽的環境以及運動員有可能是被強迫參賽的情況，或是有可能是處在非自願的選擇情況。限制運動員的自主選擇可能仍具有可行性，但這是在非常少的情況下。本文嘗試去探索一位運動醫生，在針對自主選擇的情況下所可能做的反應，如的確是自主選擇，則應在什麼樣的環境限制下所做的反應。比如，對於這樣的危險行為做反應，可能會限制運動員的行為或協助他們去比賽，這涉及到需將運動員的目標與一些美好的健康理想或醫學目的做一平衡。.

Introduction

Dealing with athletes who wish to compete in spite of a high risk of injury can be pose difficulties for sports doctors. Athletes who wish to take on such risks appear to be willing to trade good health for things they consider to be more important. The sports doctor must try to balance the aims of the athlete while safeguarding his or her health.

The primary focus of this article is to explore the obligations of doctors when responding to athletes who wish to compete at risk of injury. At times, in order to assume high levels of risk, an athlete will require medical assistance to compete. This article will explore two forms of risk assumption: those that require medical assistance and those that do not. The key questions are: Should a doctor restrict the actions of an athlete for the purposes of promoting the health of that athlete, and at what point? And should a sports doctor assist an athlete to assume high levels of risk?

At times, some of the proposed high-risk actions may result from a lack of understanding of health matters by the athlete, particularly about the potential for harm in certain situations. Many demands of athletes can be readily dealt with by education about the risks. From the literature, it appears that education about anatomy, physiology and rehabilitation matters are a large and valued part of a sports doctor's professional activities (Orchard et al. 1995, 1 – 3; Pipe 1993, 888 – 900). The individuals who are likely to cause the greatest unease in the doctor are those who, in spite of information provided by the doctor, still wish to take on what the doctor considers to be severe risks to health, and may request medical assistance to achieve this.

Limiting the Liberty of Others

It has been commonly considered that the actions of an individual should not be interfered with, particularly by the state, for the purposes of that person's own good. John Stuart Mill vigorously defended this idea:

> His own good, either physical or moral is not a sufficient warrant. He cannot be rightfully compelled to do or forbear because it will be better for him to do so, because it will make him happier, because in the opinion of others, to do so would be wise.... These are good reasons for remonstrating with him, or reasoning with him, or persuading him, or entreating him, but not for compelling him or visiting him with any evil in case he do otherwise. (Mill 1974, 68)

Feinberg explains that to force, compel or impose measures on others to protect them from harm would be to act paternalistically. Actions considered unacceptable are those 'which consist in treating adults as if they were children, or older children as if they were younger children, by forcing them to act...for their own good,...or for the good of others' (Feinberg 1986, 5). Interference in the actions of athletes will be discussed using Mill's principle and the explanations and qualifications provided by Feinberg and others.

Interference in the lives of others is generally considered to be unacceptable as it is usually considered that competent adults are able to make decisions about how they live their lives and, so long as they do not negatively impact on the lives of others, they should be left to do so. There are two reasons for this: the first is that competent adults are thought to be the best judge of their own interests; and second, it is considered that they have a right to autonomy and freedom. When others interfere in our lives it appears overbearing and patronising, generally because the implicit assumption is that in doing so they know what is best for us better than we do.

Yet this doesn't rule out paternalism completely. In fact to do so would be to 'fly in the face of both common sense and our long-established customs and laws' (Feinberg 1986, 24). There are times when even competent people have restrictions placed on them that limit actions. These may be expressed in laws requiring us to wear seatbelts or motorcycle helmets, or in prohibiting an action such as freely accessing prescription-only drugs or open access to firearms. Mill would agree with these if they can be justified in 'harm to others' terms, and this position is sometimes used. For example, it can be argued that wearing seatbelts reduces the cost to society from more serious injury. However there is potential that any law introduced to be put forward using 'harm to others' reasons when it primarily prevents harm to self (something Mill would be less than accepting of). In all of the above examples people have their liberty curtailed, and most people would say that many or all of these activities are appropriate. Support for such liberty-limiting actions can be understood as a rejection of Mill's position, at least at some level. I suggest there may indeed be times when it may be appropriate to intervene to protect someone from self-endangering harmful actions. However this does not mean that liberty-limiting interventions should be adopted freely. The underlying basis for Mill's principle of a competent person being free to live the kind of life he or she chooses is important, and so interventions into the lives of others should be minimal. The issue then becomes one of working out the circumstances in which such paternalism is justified, and understanding the implications in particular cases.

To explore the issue of risk in sport I have developed a set of cases. Each case differs from the others in a number of important ways. It is through reflection on the cases that we are able to test and develop our understanding of how we might respond. The points made about these five cases will be much more widely applicable to other similar cases.

Cases

1. An athlete, who has a contract with a professional rugby team, broke a bone in his forearm a week ago. He has been instructed not to play for six weeks to allow the fracture time to heal. He asks the sports doctor for strapping, splinting and painkillers so he can play this coming Saturday. His team is facing possible exclusion and relegation if they do not win and this athlete is clearly integral to the success of the team.
2. A top athlete facing retirement in the coming year has hip arthritis and he wants to complete his twelfth endurance race. He attends the doctor to talk about ways of minimising the pain generated by the arthritis, and to reduce excessive damage to the hip during the race. He knows that the trauma of the competition is almost certain to cause more damage to his joint surfaces with long-term effects. Despite knowing the risks he still wishes to compete.
3. An elite athlete attends the sports doctor because he has a gastro-intestinal illness that has left him with vomiting and diarrhoea for the last 48 hours. He is scheduled to run in an endurance race tomorrow for which he has trained for six months and has taken the last four months off work to compete. If he gets a placing in the top ten for this race he will be able to make the world championships, a goal he has been aspiring to for the last ten years. He will need extensive assistance to compete.
4. A batsman has just been hit on the head by a bouncing ball from a fast bowler in a cricket Test. He reels from the blow but does not fall or lose consciousness (although feels a little dizzy). A considerable bruise accompanied by swelling is apparent when he removes his helmet. He wants to continue to play.
5. A boxer received a head injury five days ago following a fall in a motorcycle accident. He was briefly knocked out and still has concussion symptoms of headache and mild visual disturbances. He wishes to compete in a match in two days' time. The sports doctor tells him about the risk of death from second impact syndrome. He decides to compete, saying that it is worth the risk.

There are some basic assumptions that need to be clarified before exploring the cases. First of all, we need to assume that all the athletes in these cases are over the age of 18. Although a number of very interesting problems arise with children in sport, the more difficult situation arises when considering limiting the actions of competent adults. The next assumption is with regard to the provision of information about risks, pathophysiology and rehabilitation. In all of these cases, it must be taken as read that these athletes have had extensive education about their injury from the sports doctor involved. In all the cases the athletes wish to play despite knowledge of the likely risks.

To stop an athlete from competing would require the doctor to take some kind of action, although it must be said that the ability to stop an athlete is limited. Such an action would probably be indirect, such as informing race or competition officials of the intended actions of the athlete and asking them to intervene to stop the athlete from competing.

In some cases, it is the doctor who is being asked to assist and presumably without such assistance the athlete would not be able to compete.

In none of these cases can it be said that the harms that could befall the athlete are in any way certain. That is, there is a chance that harm may come to the athlete, but there is always a chance the athlete will come to no harm by playing. In many ways it is the very fact that some athletes can play with an injury, despite having high risk factors for severe harm that makes this such a difficult area. Predictions of harm in sport are probabilistic.

Distinction Between Hard and Soft Paternalism

Any interference in the action of another can be understood as paternalistic. However there can be some features present within a situation that render some actions more acceptable than others. For example, we might consider it acceptable to prevent a person with severe delusions from jumping from a multi-storeyed building, whereas stopping a competent person from smoking is more difficult to justify. Here a distinction can be drawn between soft and hard paternalism. Soft paternalism can be understood as the act or practice of preventing an action by another that is considered to be harmful to that person if that action is thought to be involuntary, or when time is needed to check that this action is indeed voluntary (Feinberg 1986, 12). Actions can be thought to be involuntary from such influences as 'ignorance, coercion, derangement, drugs or other voluntary-vitiating factors' (Feinberg 1986, 5). A soft paternalist would only step in to prevent someone from carrying out an action if he or she was concerned that such action was not voluntary and harmful to the individual. Hard paternalism, on the other hand, is an action taken 'to protect competent adults against their will, from the harmful consequences even of their voluntary choices and undertakings' (Feinberg, 1986, 12). Within hard paternalism a further distinction can be made between interference on the basis that doing so would protect the ongoing capability for voluntary action of the individual and interference for other reasons.

There is some debate about whether soft paternalism is even paternalism (Feinberg, 1986, 13). Because the grounds for interference are that the action chosen by the individual is not a free and voluntary choice (for whatever reason), therefore to override such a choice is not to limit the liberty of the individual but to prevent him from acting unwittingly.

Soft Paternalist Arguments for Interference

On examination of the cases it becomes apparent that intervention may be possible in the case of the cricketer hit on the head by a fast bouncing ball (case 4) under an understanding of soft paternalism. In this case, the head injury and the signs indicate a strong possibility that this athlete has had his cognitive ability affected by a head injury. If there are such reasons for suspicions, then the doctor has good grounds for stepping in and removing the athlete from the game. This action can be justified because the sports doctor has deemed the athlete to be temporarily incompetent and therefore unable to make a reasoned assessment of his risks. If, after monitoring, the batsman is lucid and shows no signs of being affected by his head injury, soft paternalism would imply that the limitations to his action should be discontinued.

Voluntariness in Decision-making

With regard to cases 1 and 5, a soft paternalist would want to know whether there is a truly voluntary assumption of risks. Perhaps these athletes are being forced to compete against their better judgement. Because the doctor has explained the risks, it could be assumed that these athletes are making a voluntary choice. However voluntariness is not as simple as knowing the risks but is also dependent on the context in which such decision-making occurs. Athletes work in a highly contested commercial world, where there are a large number of pressures from sponsors, media and fans, creating an environment with high expectations on an athlete to succeed. In a climate where sponsorship deals are extremely lucrative but limited and where a sponsor may dictate the shoes worn and drinks consumed, it is not surprising then that the environment is set for subtle, and indeed not so subtle, pressures to be exerted on athletes to play when severe risks are present. The pressure applied to sports people differs markedly from pressures experienced by other people and many of these originate in the context of top-level sport. For example, payment structures that limit pay to playing time can make it difficult for athletes to make good choices about playing injured. The pressure from coaches and team management may also be enormous. A coach's desperation to be associated with a winning team so as to secure future coaching contracts can put excessive pressure on athletes to take risks with their health. Fear of losing a place in a team can encourage athletes to play when injured. One New Zealand All Black who played despite having had a number of head injuries states: 'There's no option. If you don't play flat out, you won't be effective, you won't be picked' (Channel Publishing group 2005, sect. 3).

The willingness of athletes to take on high levels of risk is thought to arise due to value system present in sport commonly called the 'sports ethic'. Coakley's description of the group of beliefs that make up the sports ethic can be described as:

1. An athlete makes sacrifices for 'the game'. The athlete holds 'the game' above all else and subordinates all other interests.
2. An athlete strives for distinction, aiming to improve and come closer to the goal of perfection. Coakley describes the Olympic motto *citius, altius, fortius* ('swifter, higher, stronger') as encapsulating that idea.
3. An athlete accepts risks and plays through pain, not giving in to such problems as pain or fear. There is an acceptance by the athlete of the physical risks that sport may pose to his/her health. The athlete does not shy away from challenges and to face such challenges is a sign of moral and physical bravery.
4. An athlete accepts no limits in the pursuit of possibilities. 'Real athletes' believe that sport is a sphere of life in which anything is possible if a person is dedicated enough (Coakley 1998, 153).

Sports sociologists have suggested that the sports ethic is reinforced and perpetuated by alliances between coaches and management and by sports medicine personnel (Safai 2003, 127–46). Termed 'sportsnets', these alliances are said to act in a way that normalises a culture of risk within sport. Nixon suggests that athletes who are strongly embedded within a 'sportsnet' as described above are more 'receptive to messages of risk and sacrifice and least likely to ask questions about the implications of their pain and injuries' (Nixon 1992, 127–35). So athletes are often socialised into working hard and accepting the negative consequences of such action within the context of a 'sportsnet' that expects and encourages risk taking.

But does all this mean that decisions athletes make are coerced or are in some other way non-voluntary? Coercion in its common usage describes many circumstances and situations. Wertheimer considers that for coercion to have occurred requires a threat to have been made. Offers, on the other hand, are (generally) not coercive. Threats can be understood as actions that reduce freedom, while offers increase choices and therefore freedom (Wertheimer 1987, 204). For example, if X demands that Y hand over his money or face a beating, Y's decision to hand over the money would be coerced. On the other hand, if X owned a company and offered Y a sum of money to leave a rival company and come over to work for X's company, then this would be understood as an offer and is therefore not coercive; however, there are times when offers can complicate one's decision-making, and even tempt one to blind oneself to important considerations.

So how does an understanding of the distinction between coercive and non coercive action apply to examples within sports medicine? Being offered money from a sponsor would be considered to be an offer and therefore not coercive. Pressure from fans is generally not coercive but could possibly become so – for example, if fans were to boo athletes on the field, deride them in the press or send them unpleasant mail. An athlete told by a coach to play while injured, otherwise lies would be spread about his/her work habits, would be a clear example of coercion. Other pressures such as playing with an injury for fear of losing a place in the team or not receiving a contract for the following year would not (at least at first glance) be understood as coercive.

That there are constraints on the decision-making of athletes is obvious. This, however, does not necessarily make their decisions non-voluntary or coerced. All decisions people make are to some extent constrained by something. For example, a woman with three pre-school children who decides not to have a recommended surgery because of the burdens this would place on others makes a decision that is constrained by the circumstances she finds herself in. She is making a decision that reflects the context of her own life. This does not make her decision non-voluntary or coerced but one that reflects the needs of others whom she considers are important and worthwhile to her. If an athlete decides to get involved in a contractual relationship or a sponsorship arrangement, his choices are not therefore non-voluntary, but he has committed himself to a relationship that he considers worthwhile and which place obligations on him.

Even though a threat does not exist in most instances, there are a multitude of other pressures identified above that could be making an athlete's decision less than fully voluntary. While it is clear that some instances of decision-making are voluntary and some are clearly non-voluntary, there is a large group of decisions that exist somewhere between the two. There are some times when we 'should treat voluntariness as a "variable concept," determined by higher and lower cut-off points depending on the nature of the circumstances, the interests at stake, and the moral or legal purpose to be served' (Feinberg 1986, 117). Whether a choice is voluntary or not is therefore dependent on the context the athlete finds himself in. The pressures on an athlete to keep a place in a team, to live up to expectations by fans, team members, coaches and others could create a situation where a decision is less than completely voluntary.

A case analogous to sports medicine is presented by Feinberg in his book *Harm to Self*; Lewis, a stuntman being filmed for television, is pressured into making a jump over speeding cars that ends disastrously. He does not wish to make the jump, but the director screams at him to do so, yelling 'I want you to jump now! We have a plane to catch. It's getting dark....Wrap it up, Jump!' Lewis does so and suffers severe damage to one leg, requiring amputation (Feinberg 1986, 156). While Feinberg says nobody put a gun to Lewis's head (meaning there was no overt threat) he does describe this setting as exemplifying a 'coercive climate'. Feinberg describes the shouts and taunts by the director as being 'verbal pushes and shoves' (Feinberg 1986, 158). These can be likened to a coach perhaps describing injured athletes who ask to come off the field during a game as 'wimps, who should stay on and die for the cause'. Such shouts, while not direct threats, can have a powerful effect in a situation where the athlete is tired, perhaps injured and in a state of high emotion. An athlete may also be concerned about letting people down or risking his value in the eyes of people who will be making decisions about his future. At other times the same verbal pushes and shoves would not be sufficient to negate a voluntary choice, but the combination of all of these factors would raise the question whether a decision to continue to play is voluntary enough.

Irrational or Unreasonable Choices

Some people might say that the athlete in Case Five was being unreasonable or was acting irrationally. According to Feinberg, irrational choices are those made by people who are 'retarded or deranged'. Such choices are said to be 'patently inappropriate means to his own ends, invalid deductions from his own premises, gross departures from his own ideals, or based on grotesque delusions and factual distortions. Since the deranged or retarded person is incompetent in such ways, his irrational choices are not truly his – not fully voluntary' (Feinberg 1986, 106).

Because of this we limit the claim of irrationality to those who have diminished competence. It is the competent who make unreasonable choices. Many decisions made by an athlete may appear to be irrational because they are so far from what we might choose for ourselves. We might claim that the athlete in case 5 is foolhardy or reckless because the kinds of risks he is willing to take on appear extreme and appear to run counter to his interests and goals.

Perhaps the athlete in case 5 was someone who was well known for taking risks. He may frequently drive above the speed limit or take part in the high-risk sport of base-jumping. Such a decision then could be said to fit with his character. Could we then say that a decision to compete was unreasonable? Does he require protection from such a decision? We could argue that the athlete in case 5 was making a decision in accordance with his life, an authentic choice, and while it is not a decision most would make, it is not coerced or pressured. Should he therefore be left to compete in spite of such risks and the doctor not interfere? Any interference in an effort to force him to act prudently would be to 'infringe on his autonomy' (Feinberg 1986, 109). To do so would be an act of hard paternalism. Feinberg spells out two basic rules of thumb for deciding about the self-endangering conduct of others. The first is a demand for higher levels of voluntariness when the action proposed involves high levels of risk. The second is to expect similarly high levels of voluntariness when the action involves irrevocable harm (Feinberg 1986, 117). In case 5 it appears that if this athlete accepts high levels of risk where irrevocable harm could be expected, the doctor should expect a high level of voluntariness present in the decision made by the athlete.

There are practical problems for sports doctors in assessing whether a decision is voluntary. One of the major problems that exist for the doctor in assessing voluntariness is whether the athlete feels able to discuss this with the sports doctor. The position of the sports doctor within sport might make an athlete reluctant to share information. Doctors are commonly employed by team management to care for members of the team and at times will have their loyalties divided between the coach and athlete. There may also be contractual obligations on the doctor to share medical information about an athlete with the coach and management. For a doctor to assess the voluntariness of an action, a good doctor-patient relationship would be essential to allow the athlete to confide in the doctor knowing that such information will be confidential. Sports doctors would also require a degree of independence from team management to be in a position to act in the best interests of the athlete.

To sum up so far, soft paternalism does constitute grounds for interference in the actions of another. If the athlete is in some way impaired in his/her decision-making, then the sports doctor is well placed to make such a judgement, and action to prevent the athlete from continuing or taking the field is justified. Such a decision is justified on the grounds that the athlete is not making a voluntary decision. Non-voluntary decisions can also be made by athletes who are not impaired. These decisions may not be voluntary because of coercive pressures from others such as coaches. A sports doctor should consider this possibility, but finding this out may be difficult if athletes are reluctant to confide in a doctor who has obligations to people other than the patient (Waddington and Roderick 2002, 118–23). Confidentiality would need to be assured to create an environment with the necessary trust to allow such communication to occur. Even so, assessments of coercion may be difficult to make. Judgements about whether the actions of others are voluntary (for whatever reason) are highly fallible and occasionally doctors will make decisions that are incorrect, but they would be failing in their duty if fear of making a wrong decision prevented them from interfering. Despite the potential for error, sports doctors remain ideally placed to make assessments regarding the voluntariness of an athlete's decision. This group of clinicians understand the environment of professional sport and will understand the relationships within which the athlete functions. However, doctors who identify primarily with team management may fail to recognise situations where coercion exists and may even contribute to such pressure on an athlete to play injured.

Hard Paternalist Arguments for Interference

As stated earlier, hard paternalism is interference in the voluntary actions of another. A distinction was also made between interference in actions that may threaten the future capacity for voluntary action and interference where that future capacity is not at stake. Looking again to the cases, is there ever justification for intervening in the actions of an athlete making a voluntary decision? The discussion that follows will shed light on this question.

Severity and Likelihood of Harm

To be able to make some assessment of a proposed action we would need some information about the likelihood and severity of the harms faced by the individual.

Making such an assessment is always difficult and disputes will arise even among sports doctors about how severe any harm will be and how likely it is to happen. However, in spite of this, I have attempted to assess the remaining four cases in terms of how likely and how severe the harms would be if the athlete continued with his/her planned course of action. This was done with the assistance of a senior sports doctor by placing the cases on the axis in Figure 1.

This diagram requires that some assumptions be explained. As stated earlier, all athletes are aware of the risks, and the assumption is that they are making a voluntary decision to compete. Cases 1 and 3 require a high level of physician involvement to assist the athlete to play, but risks exist even with such assistance. For example, even if the rugby player in case 1 was able to play following immobilisation of his fracture, the kind of soft immobilisation permitted on a rugby field is unlikely to afford the kind of protection such an injury would ideally need in a contact sport. Likewise, the long-distance runner who has the gastrointestinal illness will require a great deal of intravenous fluid, electrolytes and anti-nausea drugs to combat the illness and the severe dehydration in order to compete. However despite such attention, the risks associated with dehydration still exist and can escalate to such a level as to cause kidney damage and cardiac arrhythmia. Therefore a calculation of the severity and likelihood of harm is made on the basis of the athlete receiving good-quality medical care. The lines on the grid pictorially represent the gradation of severity of harm (vertical axis) from low at the bottom, to high at the top, and likelihood of harm (horizontal axis) from low (on the left) to high (on the right).[1] Because we can never say that the harms are certain, the upper end of the horizontal axis is limited to 'high' but does not reach 'certain'.

Generally the cases lie in the upper right-hand quadrant (in the right upper quadrant), indicating that these cases have the highest level of harm attached to them as well as the highest likelihood that this harm will eventuate if the athlete returns to play in

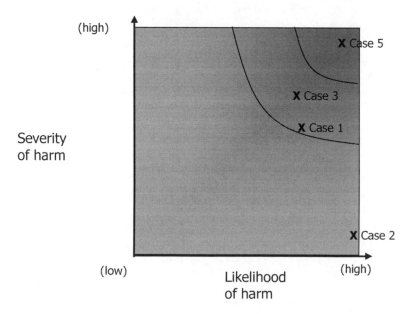

FIGURE 1
The axis of likelihood and severity of harm

the circumstances suggested in each case. This makes them the most contentious and is the reason these cases were chosen. The presence of three cases in the upper right quadrant does not simply indicate that such action should be limited but that we need to consider other factors that may make them acceptable or not.

Case 2 (the retiring endurance athlete with osteoarthritis – degenerative damage – of the hip) is the only case to lie outside the upper right quadrant on the grid. Although the likelihood of harm is high, that is, it is highly likely more damage will result to the surface of the joint; the severity of such harm is low. The race will probably only progress the damage already present in his hip, and probably to a small degree. Because the severity of harm is low, this is one example where the athlete needs to be informed about the risks involved and their likely impact on his future life and then left to make up his own mind on whether or not to proceed with such action.

I propose that any case that lay outside the upper right hand quadrant of this grid (that is, outside the right upper quadrant) should be excluded from consideration of limiting the liberty of the athlete (however, it would require that more work be done to validate and assess this in further cases). Cases that have a low likelihood of risk and a high severity (that is, cases that lie in the upper left quadrant) do not warrant intervention. These are the kinds of risks faced by any athlete who plays a contact sport or even sports such as cycling or equestrian and motor sports. There is always a risk present that something severe will happen, for example an unexpected severe head injury, or a spinal cord disruption. But events in this quadrant are generally unpredictable and unlikely; therefore any decisions about play should be left to the individual athlete. That does not mean nothing should be done, but general safeguards should be put in place to lessen those risks for the athlete; including education about risks and ensuring the use of safeguards such as mouth guards, helmets and shin guards.

Future Capacity for Voluntary Actions

Some assessment can be made to determine the nature of the harms to the athlete – for example, whether the harms are likely to involve compromising the individuals' future capacity for voluntary actions. It could be argued that harms of that kind should just be assessed as greater than other forms of harm and therefore registered further into (or towards) the right upper quadrant. However, singling out harms that compromise future capacity from other kinds of harm reminds us of the long-term and debilitating nature of such harm. In case 1 it could be argued that even if the athlete was assisted to compete and harm did eventuate, it would probably mean that the healing fracture is disrupted, or that the athlete requires surgery to fix the fracture, resulting in more time off play. His future capacity for voluntary action would not be damaged by taking to the field. In case 5, if the athlete is clearly competent and yet the outcome of a second head injury was not death but brain damage and the severe loss of cognitive function, then this would be an example of damage to that person's future capacity for voluntary action. What if an athlete voluntarily chooses to put his or her future capacity for voluntary action at risk? Remembering Feinberg's rules of thumb that insisted upon higher levels of voluntariness when the action proposed involves high levels of risk and irrevocable harm, in examining case 5 we would need to be sure that such a choice is indeed voluntary. If such a choice meets these criteria, then there may be little a doctor can do; however, this may be an area where sports governing bodies establish rules prohibiting future participation by an athlete in similar circumstances. The grounds for preventing the athlete competing could be justified in terms of harm-to-others reasoning. Killing or permanently disabling an opponent, even though that opponent had a predisposition to such an outcome, would be an unnecessary burden on the opposing athlete as well as spectators and others. If the sport was an individual sport, then preventing the athlete competing would be harder to justify.

Mitigating Factors: Importance of the Event to the Individual

We can also explore the cases for any features that may mitigate the level of risk each athlete is planning to take. One feature that may count could be the degree of planning and the significance of the event to the life plan of the athlete. The importance of the event to the individual adds weight to the decision to play because it alters our overall view of perceived benefit and harm to the athlete. It would be more difficult to justify interference in a decision where the harms were high but the athlete had been training for four years for his/her last chance at the Olympics than if the likelihood and severity of the harms were high and the athlete just wanted to compete. The net benefit to the athlete from a decision to compete will, at least to some extent, bring the level of benefits to the athlete to some comparable level with the anticipated harms that could eventuate.

Case 3 stands out as demonstrating a high level of commitment to an event. This athlete has been training for six months and given up work for the last four months in order to intensify training. He has been aspiring to making the world championships for the last ten years. Being able to compete in the event is clearly something that is important to this athlete's life plan. Compare this to the athlete in case 5 who just wishes, at risk of death following a subsequent head injury, to compete. The athlete in case 3 appears to be someone with a clearly defined goal, demonstrating a high level of planning and commitment. Despite the position on the axis, I would argue that this athlete be supported to compete. He is after all better placed than anyone else to decide what is important to him. On the other hand, this athlete has made a massive commitment to this race and it may be too difficult for him to back down and withdraw from the competition. We might want to ask questions about the likelihood of success in the race given the type of illness he has had and the requirement for an athlete performing at that level in an endurance race to perform with maximal physiological balance – something that is probably unachievable for this athlete following such an illness. It has to be said that success in achieving his goals is unlikely, but that doesn't mean he should be prevented from trying. So although case 3 falls within the right upper quadrant, the level of commitment and the importance of the event would indicate that this athlete should be supported to compete.

Indications for Intervention

When practically assessing each case, the position of the case on the axis will assist in indicating what should be done.

- Cases that fall outside of the right upper quadrant indicate that either the likelihood and/or severity of harm are low, thereby indicating that an athlete should be free to compete. However, cases in this area still require some action, including education about risks and the provision of protective gear.

- Cases that fall within the right upper quadrant would indicate the need to educate about risks, check the voluntariness of such risk assumption and determine if there are any mitigating features that could alter the assessment of net benefits.
- Cases that fall into the extreme right upper quadrant are those that indicate the highest level of both severity and likelihood of harm. These are cases that threaten an athlete's future capacity for freedom and would therefore indicate the highest level and greatest long-term risk. It is cases within this zone that could possibly warrant interference. The presence of mitigating factors in this zone would not be sufficient to alter the harm/benefit assessment. Analysis would be required on a case-by-case basis to ensure the athlete is fully aware of the implications and such a choice is free of any sort of coercive pressure, remembering that the greater the risk and more irrevocable the harm; the higher the demand for voluntariness. I would argue that cases in this region should be considered as areas where sports governing bodies may wish to establish rules that prohibit athletes from competing. Case 5 is a rare situation which would warrant such analysis.

Involvement of the Doctor in Assisting an Athlete to Take Risks

The next issue for consideration is when the doctor is asked by an athlete to assist him or her to take on high risks to health (cases 1 and 3). If an athlete requests assistance from the doctor to participate, the discussion moves from interference in the liberty of that athlete to a discussion on the duties of the doctor to act in such a way as to enhance the interests of the athlete.

How should the doctor respond to such requests? Assuming that the athlete would not be able to compete if the doctor did not assist them, some questions emerge: is the doctor in any way obligated to provide such assistance and, even if there is no obligation, should the doctor provide such assistance? Given that the doctor's skills will assist the athlete to compete and to assume severe risks, such assistance requires analysis. However, a discussion about whether the doctor should assist the athlete could not be made if the action of the athlete had been ruled out earlier. If the act proposed by the athlete had been ruled out earlier under either soft or hard paternalism, then this would mean that the doctor should not consider assisting in such a case. However because these two cases were considered not to have warranted interference on soft or hard paternalist grounds, a discussion about the duties or discretions to assist should be considered.

One of the primary issues here is how to decide between what the patient wants, what the doctor considers to be in the best interests of that patient and what is acceptable. This sets up a divided loyalty dilemma for the doctor as described by Murray:

> Physicians asked to assist someone in risking their health are in an intriguing kind of divided loyalty dilemma. They are torn between their loyalty to the patient's interests, at least as the patient defines them, and loyalty to the ends of medicine, including the pursuit of health and, not least, the renunciation of harm. (Murray 1986, 827–32)[2]

The 'ends of medicine' are not clearly defined. We might know that they exist, but dispute may exist among doctors and others about what such ends might be. Pellegrino suggests that 'medicine exists because humans become ill and want to heal, ameliorate, cure, or prevent this universal human frailty' (Pelligrino 2001, 78). The ends of medicine, according to Pellegrino, are expressed in doctor-patient relationships where decisions are made that are 'technically right' and 'morally good'. What makes a decision technically 'right' is that it is scientifically correct and in accordance with the best evidence. What makes a decision morally 'good' is that

> it is in the best interests of the patient and protects or preserves the good of the patient. The good of the patient is, in turn, a composite notion of four elements: (1) the medical good; (2) the patient's perception of his or her good; (3) the good of the patient as a human being; and (4) the spiritual good of the patient. (Pelligrino 2001, 7)

Even accepting that such ends do exist does not mean that all doctors will find them acceptable for themselves. For example a doctor may refuse to do abortions, not because he/she does not consider it a role of medicine but because he/she does not consider it acceptable to his/her own moral vision on the limits of medicine. Others may refuse on the basis that they consider this to be outside the ends of medicine.

Even if it were agreed that the ends of medicine exist and include such notions as the 'pursuit of health, and the renunciation of harm' it is difficult to know exactly whose account of harm is relevant here. What a patient might regard as harm could be very different from that of a doctor. Therefore assisting an athlete to play, at risk of harm, may well be viewed by the athlete as a good thing even when a doctor may consider that action to constitute harm. This highlights a potential conflict in Pellegrino's statement above between the medical good and the patient's perception of his or her good. It appears that there is a conflict between Murray's view and that of Pellegrino about whether such requests lie outside or inside the ends of medicine. For Murray, the patient's interest (as defined by the patient) can, at times, lie outside of the ends of medicine while Pellegrino places these interests within those ends.

While it could be considered acceptable to assist athletes at times, there should be the opportunity to refuse assistance if the doctor felt unhappy with what was being requested. In cases where athletes request assistance it is understandable that doctors would be concerned if severe harm did eventuate, as the doctor might feel some degree of responsibility for those harms. After all, if the doctor hadn't assisted the athlete the poor outcome may not have occurred as the athlete may decide not to compete. The doctor would need to consider this possibility before assisting. Conversely the opposite may happen where the athlete decides to play despite a refusal from the doctor to assist. Such action could result in a greater potential for injury; but should the doctor take any responsibility for such injury? Doctors should be able to make decisions without fear that in deciding not to assist they will be held responsible for any outcome. Such a statement would also need to be made clear to the athlete before participation and documented by the doctor.

There is a need for doctors to recognise the times when the practice of medicine (as requested by the athlete) may deviate too strongly from the ends of medicine as they are commonly understood. It is possible that doctors who identify strongly with the aims of team management may have moved too far from what is traditionally considered to be the ends of medicine. It is here that guidance from sports medicine professional bodies could provide assistance to doctors in describing acceptable medical ends and in disciplining members who have deviated too far. Doctors may also fail to recognise their own role in the production of commercialised sport, and may at times be unable to clearly identify what is in the best interest of the patient. Here again, clear guidance from the professional body can assist doctors to keep sight of the medical aims. The issue of assisting or not assisting and the implications of each action is a complex area that requires more in-depth work and analysis.

Conclusion

I have argued that intervention to prevent risk-taking in others should be taken where such action is not voluntary. After that, intervention into the actions of others should only be considered under very limited circumstances.

Threats to voluntariness can come from a number of sources including impaired cognitive function or coercive pressure. Interference in risk-taking under these circumstances is in accordance with the concept of soft paternalism. The doctor's role here is clear. If the doctor is concerned about the ability of the athlete to make an informed decision due to impaired cognition, the doctor should step in to prevent such risk-taking. When the risk of harm is extremely high, then good arguments exist for setting a higher level of voluntariness for such an action. The greatest difficulty is in finding out whether an athlete is making a truly voluntary decision. In order to know whether an athlete is voluntarily assuming risk, the sports doctor will need a close and open relationship with the athlete. Employer-employee relationships that create obligations forcing the doctor to abandon traditional obligations to the patient such as confidentiality are unlikely to encourage the athlete to speak of such concerns.

Interference on hard paternalist lines should be limited to rare circumstances. If a doctor is concerned about the level of risk, the first response should be education about risks. After this, if the athlete still wants to take on such risks, interference should be limited to those situations where the likelihood and severity of harm is high and where the future capacity for voluntary action is threatened. I argue that only in these rare circumstances would it be acceptable for doctors to intervene.

When an athlete requests assistance from a doctor to play where high levels of risk exist, and where participation would be impossible without such assistance, the doctor would need to consider a number of issues. These issues include whether the doctor is willing to comply, given the injury that could result: is this something he or she is willing to accept? The answer relates to whether the doctor considers such a request is within the ends of medicine. Assistance with this question could be given some consideration by the professional body in order to offer some guidance to sports doctors.

ACKNOWLEDGEMENTS
The author is grateful for the assistance of Andrew Moore, David Gerrard, Neil Pickering, Claire Gallop and Mike King.

NOTES

1. The two separate axis originated from Feinburg 1986.
2. There has been some discussion about whether the ends of medicine should be understood as being intrinsic to its very nature or whether they are socially constructed (see Wertheimer 1987, 204). The ends Murray mentions are very like those Pellegrino attributes to an intrinsic view.

REFERENCES

ANON. 2005. Heading for recovery. *Healthwise*, June/July: 3.

COAKLEY, J. 1998. *Sport in Society*. 6th edn. Boston, MA: McGraw-Hill.

FEINBERG, J. 1986. *Harm to Self*. New York: Oxford University Press.

MILL, J.S. 1974. *On Liberty*. London: Penguin Books.

MURRAY, T. 1986. Divided loyalties for physicians: Social context and moral problems. *Social Science and Medicine* 23 (8): 827 – 32.

NIXON, H. 1992. A social network analysis of influences on athletes to play with pain and injuries. *Journal of Sport and Social Issues* 16 (2): 127 – 35.

ORCHARD, J., P. FRICKER and P. BRUKNER. 1995. Sports medicine for professional teams. *Clinical Journal of Sport Medicine* 5: 1 – 3.

PELLEGRINO, E. 2001. Professional codes. In *Methods in Medical Ethics*, edited by J Sugarman and D Sulmasy. Washington, DC: Georgetown University Press: 314.

PIPE, A. 1993. Sport, science, and society: Ethics in sports medicine. *Medicine and Science in Sports and Exercise* 25 (8): 888 – 900.

SAFAI, P. 2003. Healing the body in the 'culture of risk': Examining the negotiation of treatment between sports medicine clinicians and injured athletes in Canadian intercollegiate sport. *Sociology of Sport Journal* 20: 127 – 46.

WADDINGTON, I. and M. RODERICK. 2002. Management of medical confidentiality in English professional football clubs: Some ethical problems and issues. *British Journal of Sports Medicine* 36: 118 – 23.

WERTHEIMER, A. 1987. *Coercion*. In *Studies in Moral, Political and Legal Philosophy*, edited by Marshall Cohen. Princeton, NJ: Princeton University Press.

DOPING UNDER MEDICAL CONTROL – CONCEPTUALLY POSSIBLE BUT IMPOSSIBLE IN THE WORLD OF PROFESSIONAL SPORTS?

Søren Holm

This paper considers the argument that if the ban on doping in sports was abolished it would be possible to have doping under medical control, i.e. open doping, prescribed by doctors with collection of reliable information about effects and side-effects. A game-theoretic argument is developed showing that this positive scenario is very unlikely to be instantiated given reasonable assumptions about the motivation of sportspersons and sports doctors. It is furthermore shown that the standard arguments against the current ban on doping also entail that if doping was made legal any requirements that it should be open doping could not be justified.

Resumen

Este artículo considera el argumento de que si la prohibición sobre el dopaje en los deportes fuese suprimida sería posible el tener dopaje bajo supervisión médica, esto es, dopaje sin trabas, prescrito por doctores con una recolección de información fiable acerca de los efectos y los efectos secundarios. Se desarrolla un argumento teórico del juego mostrando que este cuadro positivo es muy poco probable que se dé dadas suposiciones razonables acerca de la motivación de los deportistas y los médicos del deporte. Adicionalmente se demuestra que los argumentos comunes contra la presente prohibición sobre el dopaje también implican que si el dopaje ha de ser legalizado cualquier requerimiento de que debería de ser dopaje sin trabas no podría ser justificado.

Zusammenfassung

Dieser Aufsatz befasst sich mit der Behauptung, dass es im Falle der Aufhebung des Dopingverbots möglich sei, Doping von medizinischer Seite kontrollieren zu können, d.h. Dopingfreigabe bei ärztlicher Kontrolle und somit Überwachung der Effekte und Nebeneffekte. Mit Hilfe der Spieltheorie lässt sich begründen, warum dieses positive Szenario, unter Berücksichtigung begründeter Annahmen über die Motivation von Sportlern und Sportärzten, sehr unwahrschein-lich ist. Des Weiteren lässt sich zeigen, dass die gängigen Argumente der Befürworter einer Dopingfreigabe, sowie die Anforderungen an ein offenes Doping sich nicht rechtfertigen lassen.

摘要

本文考慮到一個論點：假如運動禁藥措施解禁的話，那這樣就有可能用醫學方法來控管禁藥，也就是說禁藥在開放的同時也受到專業醫師依據可靠醫藥資訊來提供處方。用一種遊戲理論的主張可顯示出這樣的美好場景不太可能產生，這是因為運動參與者與運動醫生的動機理由。 進一步來說，現行反對運動禁藥的一些標準主張也同時包括： 假如運動禁藥合法的話，那就開放它的各種需求主張是不能夠被證成接受的。

Introduction

One of the arguments in the debate about whether or not the current blanket ban on doping in sports should be lifted is that if the ban is lifted it will be possible to have doping under medical control. If doping becomes legitimate there is no longer a need for sportspersons to hide that they are using doping and no longer a need for doctors to hide that they are prescribing doping.[1] This would, according to the argument, entail a number of positive consequences: (1) that the sportsperson can access impartial medical advice about the effectiveness and side-effects of different doping methods and can therefore make a more informed decision; (2) that side-effects of doping are picked up more quickly and dealt with more effectively; and (3) that it will be possible to collect reliable information about the effects and side-effects of different doping techniques because sportspersons and sports doctors will be able to share their experiences. (Kayser et al. 2005).

In this paper I will critically analyse this argument and show that it is very unlikely that these positive effects will occur as a general phenomenon across all, or even most, sports and doping techniques. I will mainly focus the analysis on the situation facing the professional sportsperson, but some of the arguments and conclusions will also apply to non-professional sportspersons who are part of, for instance, national teams.

The argument that the lifting of the ban on doping will lead to safe doping under medical control is usually not the main argument put forward to justify changing the doping rules. The main arguments are usually either liberal/libertarian, conventionalist or consistency arguments, or some combination of these (Spriggs 2005, 112–13; Tännsjö 2005, 113; Tamburrini 2000; 2006). The liberal/libertarian arguments claim that unless doping can be shown to harm other people than the people doping themselves it should not be prohibited in a liberal society, since prohibition would then be paternalistic. The conventionalist arguments point out that the rules of sports are conventions and that they therefore ought to reflect what really happens in the sport, not what outsiders would ideally want to happen. So if active sportspersons regularly take doping substances, that should be allowed by the rules. And finally the consistency arguments rely on showing that we cannot draw a line between doping and other performance-enhancing activities and procedures in sport (e.g. no justifiable line between EPO use and the use of hypoxic air machines or high-altitude training). These arguments are not analysed in this paper, but as we shall see they constrain what actions we can justify to ensure that legal doping is also safe doping under medical control.

Some Initial Distinctions

Initially it is necessary to make some distinctions concerning different sports and different doping techniques. Sport is usually defined as 'institutionalized competitive activities that involve vigorous physical exertion or the use of relatively complex physical skills by individuals whose participation is motivated by a combination of internal and external factors' (Coakley 1994, 21). [4]

But, as we are all aware, this leaves a very large range of human activities within the concept of sport, and a huge range of distinctions can be applied to this set of activities. The distinctions that are important here are not so much distinctions concerning the different types of sports but distinctions concerning the contexts in which sports take place and professional sportspersons are employed, because those contexts influence their ability to act in relation to doping.

The first important distinction is a distinction concerning the degree to which the sportsperson is employed and controls his or her income stream. Is the sportsperson self-employed with income mainly from prize money, self-employed with income mainly from sponsorship, employed but with income mainly from sponsorship or employed with income mainly from the employer? (Similar distinctions apply to sportspersons who are technically amateurs but who sustain their sports activities by income generated by these activities.)

The second distinction concerns the degree of control the sportsperson has over the decision to play. Does the sportsperson have personal control over both the decision to play, and the decision not to play in a given instance?[2] There are in reality two issues here. The first is an issue of formal control. In many team sports a considerable degree of control over who plays is exercised by the coach of the team, or a committee of selectors. The same is the case for a number of individual sports where a sportsperson is only allowed to compete if chosen by his or her association. In these cases the sportsperson can decide not to play, but he or she cannot decide to play if he/she is not selected. The second is an issue of informal control: 'stars' may well be able to demand to play, and sportspersons may, on the other hand, also be leaned upon to compete even if they don't want to.

The third distinction concerns the degree of control the sportsperson has over the choice of medical adviser and the medical adviser's employment status.[3] Is the medical adviser chosen and employed by the sportsperson, or is he or she chosen and employed by the sportspersons' employer?

We also need to make distinctions concerning different forms of doping. I will here mainly focus on doping with pharmaceutically active substances, but I think the arguments can be extended to other forms of doping techniques as well. We can distinguish between:

1. Well known drugs with well known doping effects (e.g. beta-adrenergic antagonists for the removal of hand tremor in shooting sports);
2. Well-known drugs with not generally known doping effects;
3. Well-known drugs with doping effects outside the normal clinical dosing range;[4]
4. Experimental drugs developed by the mainstream pharmaceutical industry; and
5. Experimental drugs developed outside the mainstream pharmaceutical industry.

Legal Doping and Impartial Advice in the Triangle of Death and Injury

Let us consider the average professional footballers (i.e. soccer players), rugby players or handball players. They will be on contract with a specific club and will usually play when, but only when, the coach says so. Their main income will be from the club, and although they will be earning well, they will not be able to build up savings that will allow them to walk away from the game before late in their career, if ever.[5] Their medical adviser will be a doctor employed by the club.[6] They will thus have the least personal control over their situation and their adviser of any professional sportsperson, according to the distinctions drawn above. Many other sportspersons on national teams receiving personal sponsorship from the national sports organisation will be in an essentially similar situation.

In this case we have a triangle with the employer, the sportsperson and the sports doctor at each corner (see Figure 1), although the employer's influence on the sportsperson is often mediated through the team coach or manager.

Within this triangle it is worth considering to what degree the sports doctor acts or can act as the agent of the sportsperson or to what degree he or she acts or will have to act as (at least partially) the agent of the employer. There are numerous examples of players who have been given dangerous treatments for injuries, or told to play despite injury, in the interest of the team winning, without being told what the real risk were. This indicates that at least some sports doctors do act as agents for their employers, even when this is of detriment to their patients.[7]

If the sports doctor is rational, and unencumbered by adherence to the traditional ethical standards of the medical profession or the newer ethical standards of sports medicine, it is also easy to see that this is the decision he or her must rationally make. A sports doctor who knows on which side his bread is buttered will also know that stable employment often requires that one does not act in ways that are too contrary to the interests of the principal. The sportsperson could of course go elsewhere to get a second

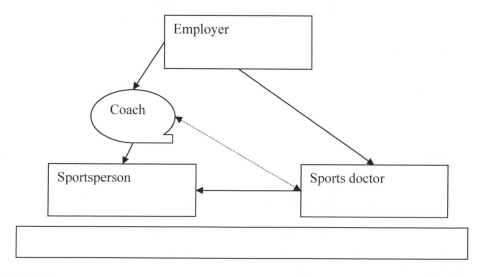

FIGURE 1
The relation between sportspersons and other relevant parties

opinion, but he or she would often be forced to follow the club doctor's advice even if it was problematic.

This means that even if doping became legal and sports doctors could therefore legitimately advise sportspersons about doping methods, their effects and their side-effects, we should not expect sports doctors to provide impartial advice if they, and the sportspersons they advise, are in the position outlined above.

If the sportsperson is living off prize money and employing his or her own advisers the situation will be different. In that case the advisers will have no interest in offering partial advice, and may even have a positive interest in giving impartial advice.[8] Truly independent sportspersons will therefore be able to get impartial advice if doping became legal, but this would not be the case for most professional sportspersons.

Remaining Competitive in an Era of Legal Doping

Let us imagine that the ban on doping has been lifted and I am a sportsperson who is being given the option of using a new experimental drug developed by the best sports pharmacologists the nation can afford. I am told that it can probably boost my performance significantly but that its side-effects are not known, since it is just out of the laboratory. It does, however, not seem to be particularly harmful to the rats and mice it has been tested on.

Because I am known to be a person of good judgement I am also told that I can decide whether or not the existence of this drug should be made public, and it should be provided to other sportspersons who want it.

What should I do? If I want to gain and maintain a competitive advantage, and it is probably safe to assume that I do given the huge amounts of training I am and have been putting in, it will in many circumstances be rational for me to ask that the existence of the drug be kept secret. As long as the drug is a secret my competitors will not have access to it and I can keep my advantage. I may realise that this will not last forever – someone is sure to find out at some point (although the risks of that must decrease if there are no doping controls) – but that is irrelevant to the rationality of my decisions as long as I get a reasonable spell of exclusive use.[9]

If I thought that there was a high risk of side-effects, it would change the rationality of my decision, since knowledge about side-effects and how to deal with them could be generated much faster if more people took the drug; but then a high risk of side-effects would make my decision to take the drug in the first place of questionable rationality.[10]

If we formalise the situation, we can see that it is a classic game-theoretical problem, where the option to 'take and hide' dominates the other options under reasonable assumptions about effects and side-effects; and furthermore that if we reject that option, 'reject and hide' becomes the dominant option. It is thus only if the pay-off matrix is changed that it becomes rational to choose to take the doping substance openly. If a sportsperson was driven by a motive of general benevolence, or adhered to a strictly utilitarian calculus, 'reject and hide' would again be the dominant option in a condition of imperfect compliance (i.e. if not everyone is generally benevolent) or if 'trembling hand' considerations apply so that some might take the drug (e.g. because of weakness of will), and it would only be in ideal theory that 'reject and tell' would become dominant, since no one would desert from the common optimum to seek their individual optimum.

We can therefore conclude that in a situation where the ban on doping is dropped, the positive 'publicity' consequences are unlikely to occur in any situation where the drug

TABLE 1
Game theoretical analysis of the openness of legitimate doping

Option	Take and hide	Take and tell	Reject and hide	Reject and tell
Consequences for the sportsperson	Competitive advantage, but larger risk of untreatable side-effects	Competitive status quo, with lower risk of untreatable side-effects	Competitive status quo, no side-effects	Competitive disadvantage, no side-effects
Consequences for other sportspersons	Competitive disadvantage, no side-effects	Competitive status quo, with lower risk of untreatable side-effects	Competitive status quo, no side-effects	Competitive advantage, with lower risk of untreatable side-effects

Note: This analysis is under the assumption that if the drug becomes known a significant number of competitors will take it.

itself, or the doping effect of the drug, can be kept secret by those who first discover or use it. We should therefore expect to see open use of well-known drugs with well-known doping effects, but hidden use of other doping methods.

If doping effects varied between athletes, for instance according to some genetic factor, we might expect the game-theoretical calculations to become more complicated. And so they are, but not hugely so. There is only one situation in which differential effect can make 'take and tell' the rational option, and that is if the sportsperson has a high degree of certainty that he or she will be at the top end of the differential effectiveness scale. Although this situation is unlikely to occur, it will make 'take and tell' slightly more likely than it would otherwise be, but it would conversely also make the two 'hide' options slightly more prevalent, since the sportsperson knowing that he or she was at the lower end of the differential effectiveness would have a stronger incentive to hide the knowledge about the substance.

If I was employed by a club or on a national team in a situation as described above it is probably highly unlikely that I would be given the choice. From the employer's point of view the 'take and hide' option is even more dominant because it is unlikely that the full costs of any side-effects will fall on the employer. Few handball clubs for instance compensate, or have to compensate, their retired players for the damaged joints resulting from an often too early return to competitive sport after the first knee injury.

Bring Back the Good Doctor?

Two possibilities might be suggested to avoid the negative conclusions reached above concerning the positive effects of legal doping. We could impose, or perhaps more accurately re-impose, obligations on sports doctors to act as exclusive agents for the individual sportsperson. Or we could impose obligations on both sportspersons and sports doctors to be fully open concerning their doping practices. The latter of these options, if enforced with suitable punishments for non-compliance constitute an adjustment to the pay-offs in our game, imposing a penalty for the 'hide' option.

The first of these options would essentially amount to reaffirming the traditional obligation of the medical doctor not to act against the interests of his or her patient as it is for instance expressed in a large number of oaths and declarations. The World Medical Association's International Code of Medical Ethics states that:

> A PHYSICIAN SHALL not permit motives of profit to influence the free and independent exercise of professional judgement on behalf of patients.

> A PHYSICIAN SHALL in all types of medical practice, be dedicated to providing competent medical service in full technical and moral independence, with compassion and respect for human dignity.

> A PHYSICIAN SHALL deal honestly with patients and colleagues, and strive to expose those physicians deficient in character or competence, or who engage in fraud or deception....

> A PHYSICIAN SHALL owe his patients complete loyalty and all the resources of his science. Whenever an examination or treatment is beyond the physician's capacity he should summon another physician who has the necessary ability.[11]

And The Code of Ethics of Sports Medicine Australia holds that members shall

- Uphold the mission of Sports Medicine Australia.
- Respect human life and well being....
- *Provide an objective and confidential service to the best of his/her ability – with the sports person's best interests in mind.*
- Show prudence and balanced judgements when dealing with any situation that may confront them, whilst upholding the mission of Sports Medicine Australia.
- Never deny attention to any sports person on the basis of their culture, ethnicity, religion, political beliefs, sex, sexual orientation or the nature of their injury or condition.
- Inform and advise the sports person about the nature of their injury or condition and its possible consequences, the probable cause and available treatments or programs with the likely benefits and risks of each....
- Make available, any knowledge acquired through further study or other avenues, for the benefit of all.[12]

If we could successfully enforce such an obligation the sportsperson would at least be offered impartial advice, and would thus be in a better position to make informed decisions concerning doping. We would not, however, have ensured any better reporting of doping use, effects and side-effects.

The second option would require us to impose a new obligation, but would probably be more effective if it could be enforced. It would make it possible to collect complete information about doping use, effects and side-effects and make this information available to all sportspersons and sports doctors. As long as there is some advantage in hidden doping we can, however, only expect compliance with a reporting obligation if there are ways of catching and punishing the cheats (i.e. those who do not report as they ought to). To ensure compliance with a reporting obligation we will therefore need doping control, bringing us back to square one.

There is also another problem with these two suggestions. Neither of them are available to most of the philosophers who advocate an end to the doping ban, if they want to avoid inconsistency.

Most of the philosophers who argue against the ban on doping do so from premises that are either strongly conventionalist or strongly libertarian, or in many cases a mix of these.

One prominent type of conventionalist argument is that the ethics of a sport is what the players of the sport say it is, either in their verbal statements or in their actions on the playing field. It is thus only if the players want a ban on doping, and do not regularly engage in doping, that such a ban is justified. It cannot be imposed because of some abstract notion of the ethics (or essence) of the sport held by, for instance, the sport's governing body. The governing body is almost never composed of those who are currently active in the sport and thus lacks the legitimacy to impose rules on those who are active, according to the conventionalist argument. But it is rather obvious that an exactly parallel argument can be made with regard to sports doctors. The ethics of sports doctoring is what sports doctors say it is etc. If sports doctors in a particular sport therefore regularly put the interest of the team, or the interests of their employer above the interests of the individual player who is their patient, that is how it should be, and they should not be forced to change just because outsiders have other views concerning this ethical issue.[13]

The libertarian line of argument is also, as most libertarian arguments, rather simple.[14] Unless it can be shown that some action I want to take is directly harmful to others – and both libertarians and liberals often operate with rather narrow conceptions of what constitutes a harm – it is unethical to prevent me from performing the action if I want to, even if it is harmful to myself. If I want to take doping that is my decision, unless it can be shown that my action is directly harmful to others. A subsidiary line of argument points out that doping control in itself constitutes and infringement of liberty.

This may seem to give us a reason to require doctors to be impartial since partial advice may harm the recipient. But it would not give us a reason to impose this obligation on doctors who do not hold themselves out to be impartial. If my patients know that I am not their agent, and ask for my advice anyway, I do not harm them by giving them partial advice.[15] *Volenti non fit injuria*. That they may be somewhat coerced by another agent to use me as an adviser is not my problem.

And the libertarian argument even more strongly undermines any reason to require openness about doping. If no one is harmed by doping in the current situation where doping is illegal, and accordingly rather secretive, it is very hard to see how they could be damaged if someone kept his or her doping secret in a context where doping was legitimate. If secret doping does not constitute cheating now, it could not constitute cheating if doping was legalised.

Safe Drugs for Doping?

A further issue is whether legalisation of doping will lead to drugs for doping being tested more thoroughly than they are currently before they are used by sportspersons. Will the pharmaceutical industry have an interest in developing and testing doping substances, and will sportspersons have an interest in waiting to use the substances until they can be marketed under current regulatory standards for drugs or nutritional supplements?

Whether the pharmaceutical industry will have an interest in developing and testing completely new doping substances almost exclusively depends on the size of the market, and thereby probably on (1) whether these substances can also be successfully marketed to non-elite sportspersons, or (2) whether they have non-doping uses. If doping became legitimate we would probably see firms studying and promoting the doping effects of drugs they had developed for other purposes, but it is unclear whether a drug whose sole use was for doping could ever economically repay the very large investment necessary to develop it so that it could be registered according to current regulatory standards. The only exception being drugs that would be of benefit to both elite and non-elite sportspersons across a range of sports, for instance drugs that speed up recovery after injury. It is therefore likely that many promising (or tempting) doping substances will not be registered as pharmaceutical specialties or nutritional supplements, and furthermore that it will become evident to inventors or producers of these substances very early on in the development process that it does not make economic sense to perform the necessary testing, because it will be impossible ever to recoup the investment. This does, however, not mean that the substances cannot be sold as pure chemicals and used by sportspersons, just that they will be untested and that the producers cannot refer to their possible doping effects in any way. A regulator might well find this an unsafe and unsatisfactory state of affairs and try to ban the sale of such substances if there is evidence of misuse (i.e. any use by human beings). It is therefore likely that a range of doping substances will still be illegal to sell, even if the practice of doping itself becomes legal.

But now our libertarian interlocutor will be eager to put forward an objection that goes to the second part of our question above, and which is almost identical to the original objection concerning the prohibition of doping in sport. It is fairly obvious that elite sportspersons may have an interest in using a doping substance long before it has reached the high standard of evidence concerning safety and efficacy that is necessary to have it formally registered as a drug, especially if this means that their competitors are less likely to use it (e.g. because of lack of knowledge about its effects, or lack of access). If the sportsperson thinks that the risk is worth taking in order to increase the chances of a good performance, what would the justification be for intervening? Would an intervention not be pure paternalism? Yes, an intervention would be pure paternalism, but it might be the only way to ensure safe doping procedures.

We have therefore again come up against an impasse in the argument. We can only have the good effects of doping under medical control if we continue to restrict the actions of sportspersons and sports doctors. The restrictions will be different than the restrictions we have now when doping is illegal, but they will still not allow the sportsperson to take any doping substance he wants to take in the way he or she wants to take them. Only open doping can be allowed, and this would require the continuation of doping control to detect those who cheat by hiding their doping use.

Conclusion

In this paper I have shown that we have no reason to believe that the legalisation of doping will lead to a situation where open doping under medical control will become the norm. This means that one of the alleged positive effects of legalising doping is unlikely to occur.

This does not show that doping should not be legalised, but just that we should not expect the world of sports to become a much better place if it is, or doping a much safer practice.

NOTES

1. I use the slightly artificial term 'sportsperson', not primarily because it is gender-neutral, but because it is neutral between different sports. It does not, as the term 'athlete', have connotations of athletics and/or individual competition. Lifting the ban on doping would presumably also make it legitimate for firms producing doping substances to market these for their doping effects under similar rules to the marketing of other pharmacologically active substances.

2. I include those sports where the right to compete in a given tournament is decided according to a transparent merit system, such as tennis and golf (apart from the existence of wild cards), in the group of sports where a sportsperson can have full personal control over the decision to play.

3. The choice and the employment issues can obviously be disentangled, but since they very often go together I do not think that it is necessary to introduce a further distinction here.

4. This group also include those drugs that are no longer in clinical use, like most anabolic steroids. Our medical knowledge about such drugs varies enormously depending mainly on the time span during which they were in clinical use.

5. Note that the average Premier League or Serie A player is not the average professional player in economic terms. Income in the lower leagues is much less than in the top leagues. Whereas the average wage for an English Premier League player was £676,000 in 2005, it was less than £50,000 in the old fourth division (now 'League Two'). See '£676,000: The average salary of a Premiership footballer in 2006', *The Independent* (London), 11 April 2006, available at http://sport.independent.co.uk/football/news/article357006.ece, accessed 23 November 2006.

6. They may also receive health advice from the club's physiotherapist, masseur, sports psychologist, nutritionist and so on, but to simplify I will here only consider the doctor.

7. The same phenomenon is well documented for coaches who are also supposed to have the best interests of the sportspersons they coach as their main concern. Whereas we may not think that coaches in professional sports should always prioritise the interests of the individual sportsperson, even when that interest is an interest in life and limb, it is generally believed that coaches of young sportspersons should prioritise the health interests of their charges, but even with regard to young athletes there are many examples of coaches prioritising other interests.

8. Unless the sportspersons become so rich, famous and self-important that advisers just tell them what they want to hear.

9. That is, for instance, also the reason that certain business secrets (and drinks recipes e.g. for Coca-Cola and Drambuie) are kept as proprietary information and not patented, which would make them public.

10. I am here assuming that we can simplify the problem and consider only the involved sportspersons. This is probably a reasonable assumption in most cases, but we can

imagine situations where the general elation if a certain record is broken or a certain achievement is achieved will be so great that it could make the 'take and tell' option the option preferred in a utilitarian calculus because it increases the chance that the record will be broken, and many people made happy.

11.   World Medical Association International Code of Medical Ethics.

12.   Sports Medicine Australia Code of Ethics.

13.   This kind of conventionalist argument occurs in many discussions about whether something (X) is a practice that doctors should be involved in (e.g. plastic surgery or abortion). Opponents say that X is outside medicine, but proponents counter that medicine is what doctors (and perhaps society) makes it.

14.   In the doping debate it is often difficult to distinguish libertarians from liberals since the arguments against the ban on doping mainly concern a right to be free from restrictions, an area where liberal and libertarian arguments concur.

15.   This is simply a version of the well-known doctor/schmoktor argument. There may be special ethical rules for doctors, but if I am a schmoktor and everyone knows that, there is no reason why I should be bound by the rules for doctors.

REFERENCES

COAKLEY, JAY J. 1994. *Sport in Society: Issues and Controversies.* New York: McGraw-Hill.

KAYSER, B., A. MAURON and A. MIAH. 2005. Viewpoint: Legalisation of performance-enhancing drugs. *The Lancet* 366 (1): S21.

SPORTS MEDICINE AUSTRALIA. Code of Ethics. Available at http://www.sma.org.au/about/ethics.asp, accessed 23 November 2006.

SPRIGGS, M. 2005. Hypoxic air machines: Performance enhancement through effective training – or cheating? *Journal of Medical Ethics* 31: 112–13.

TAMBURRINI, C.M. 2000. *The 'Hand of God'? Essays in the Philosophy of Sports.* Göteborg: Acta Universitatis Gothoburgensis.

———. 2006. Are doping sanctions justified? A moral relativistic view. *Sport in Society* 9 (2): 199–211.

TÄNNSJÖ, T. 2005. Hypoxic air machines – commentary. *Journal of Medical Ethics* 31: 113.

WORLD MEDICAL ASSOCIATION. International Code of Medical Ethics. Adopted by the 3rd General Assembly of the World Medical Association, London, England, October 1949, and amended by the 22nd World Medical Assembly, Sydney, Australia, August 1968 and the 35th World Medical Assembly, Venice, Italy, October 1983.

GENETICS, BIOETHICS AND SPORT

Andy Miah

This paper considers the relevance of human genetics as a case study through which links between bioethics and sport ethics have developed. Initially, it discusses the science of gene-doping and the ethics of policy-making in relation to future technologies, suggesting that the gene-doping example can elucidate concerns about the ethics of sport and human enhancement more generally. Subsequently, the conceptual overlap between sport and bioethics is explored in the context of discussions about doping. From here, the paper investigates the ethics of gene-doping, arguing that a straightforward mapping of medical ethics onto sport ethics is not justified. In conclusion, it argues that gene-doping is consistent with a broader ethics of enhancement within elite sports. Moreover, the increased legitimacy of lifestyle medicine in society is likely to reduce the relevance of an anti-doping programme that is concerned with protecting the integrity of an alleged natural athlete.

Resumen

Este artículo considera la relevancia de la genética humana como un caso de estudio a través del cual pueden desarrollarse conexiones entre la bioética y la ética deportiva. Inicialmente presenta la ciencia del dopaje de los genes y la ética de la creación de pólíticas al respecto en relación a tecnologías futuras, sugiriendo que el ejemplo del dopaje de genes puede despejar precupaciones acerca de la ética deportiva y el amejoramiento físico humano en general. A continuación, el campo conceptual común entre deporte y bioética es explorado en el contexto de debates acerca del dopaje. En conclusión, argumenta que el dopaje de genes es consistente con una ética más amplia del amejoramiento dentro de la élite. Además, la creciente legitimidad de la medicina sobre el modo de vida en la sociedad es probable que reduzca la importancia de un programa anti-dopaje que se preocupe de la protección de la integridad de un supuesto atleta natural.

Zusammenfassung

Dieser Aufsatz sieht in der Humangenetik ein geeignetes Fallbeispiel zur Darstellung der Verbindungslinien zwischen Bioethik und Sportethik. Zunächst soll das Feld Gendoping und die Ethik der politischen Entscheidungsfindung, im Hinblick auf Zukunftstechnologien im Zentrum der Diskussion stehen. Hierbei wird unterstellt, dass das Beispiel Gendoping zum einen, sowohl die sportethischen Bedenken, als auch die Fragen nach Leistungssteigerung des Menschen im Allgemeinen, verdeutlichen kann. Anschließend werden im Rahmen der Dopingdiskussion die theoretischen Anknüpfungspunkte zwischen Sport und Bioethik untersucht. Des Weiteren analysiert dieser Artikel die ethischen Implikationen des Gendopings, wobei behauptet wird, dass die direkte Übertragung der Medizinethik auf die Sportethik nicht gerechtfertigt ist. Schließlich wird argumentiert, dass Gendoping in einem weiten Ethikverständnis konsistent ist mit der Bewertung der Leistungssteigerung im Leistungsport. Nicht zuletzt wird durch die steigende Akzeptanz der Lifestyle Medizin in der Gesellschaft die Bedeutung der Anti-Doping Maßnahmen wahrscheinlich abnehmen. Denn jene Maßnahmen haben zum Ziel die Integrität des vermeintlich natürlichen Athleten zu schützen.

摘要

本文將人類基因視為一個個案研究，將生物倫理學及已發展的運動倫理學聯結起來。首先，探討的是基因禁藥科學和未來科技相關政策決定之倫理學，而指出基因禁藥的範例，可以更具一般性地闡釋關於運動倫理學以及提高人類能力的課題。接著，探討了運動與生物倫理學之間重疊的部份。本文調查了基因禁藥的倫理學，認為直接將醫學倫理學套用在運動倫理學的做法，是值得爭議的。本文的結論提出，基因禁藥的課題，和存在於優秀運動員內部的廣泛的倫理學課題是一致的。進一步而言，社會生活中逐漸增加的醫學合法性，很可能會減少了反禁藥計畫的措施，這個措施是與保護宣稱合乎自然的運動員之純潔性是有關聯的。

Introduction

In the last five years, the application of gene transfer technology to sport has gained the attention of many sporting and non-sporting institutions around the world. In 2001, the International Olympic Committee (IOC) Medical Commission convened a working group to examine the emerging applications of gene therapy for sport (International Olympic Committee 2001). During the same year, the Australian Law Reform Commission (ALRC) published a draft paper on the legal implications of using genetic information, one section of which is devoted to sport (Australia Law Reform Commission 2001). In 2002, the World Anti-Doping Agency met at the Cold Spring labs in Banbury, New York, in the first of its discussions on how genetic technology might be used for doping. As well, the United States President's Council on Bioethics held two meetings where sport was a focus for their discussion (US President's Council on Bioethics 2002a; 2002b). In 2003, the American Association for the Advancement of Science held a symposium on the science and ethics of gene technology and sport (AAAS 2003). Further, the ALRC published its final report, *Essentially Yours,*' which highlights sport as a key area of concern. In February 2004, the AAAS met again to discuss the matter (Kane 2004) alongside new research from growth-factor gene scientist Lee Sweeney, whose publication in the March edition of the *Journal of Applied Physiology* (Lee et al. 2004) suggests further how gene-doping might arise. Also, the Netherlands Centre for Doping Affairs and the World Anti-Doping Agency held another workshop on gene doping, this time in the Netherlands.[1] Some scientists even speculated that genetically modified athletes might be present at the Athens 2004 Olympic Games. Most recently, WADA held its second landmark meeting on Gene Doping, where it developed its 'Stockholm Declaration' (World Anti-Doping Agency 2005). One of the major outcomes of this meeting was to urge against the use of genetic tests in sport, at a time when the first commercial test for performance genes had just been made available: '7. The use of genetic information to select for or discriminate against athletes should be strongly discouraged. This principle does not apply to legitimate medical screening or research.'

This all takes place now in a climate of greater uncertainty about the role of anti-doping in elite sport. As a further threat to WADA's aspirations, towards the end of 2003, a syringe filled with unknown designer steroid tetrahydrogestrinone (THG) caused concern in the sports world when it was left anonymously at Don Catlin's international doping lab at UCLA. This occurrence reinforced the concern that anti-doping tests continue to lag behind the many number of possible methods athletes are actually using to alter their performances. For many, gene-doping might soon be one of those methods, and the desire for WADA to ensure it is ahead of the 'cheaters' is central to why these discussions are taking place now.

This paper argues that gene-doping will make explicit the inadequacies of the ethical foundation of anti-doping policy, which demand that it cannot be construed as merely another form of doping. Additionally, by opening up the anti-doping debate to broader bioethical concerns, gene-doping provides a case whereby a more informed and rigorous approach to establishing what is valuable about sport can develop. Indeed, at present, anti-doping rests firmly on a restrictive application of medical ethical principles. This approach has omitted to utilise the academic literature in the philosophy of sport, which has developed over the past 30 years (alongside but separate from the same development in bioethics) as well as critical positions in bioethics. The paper first presents an overview of the science of gene-doping with an initial response to the concerns that discussion about this matter should not be taken seriously. It then explores the rich connections that exist between bioethics and sport ethics, which suggest fruitful links between these two areas of research. Subsequently, a review of the gene doping debate is provided followed by a response and proposal for how the discussion might be best advanced.

The Science of Gene Doping

The scientific perspective on possibility of gene-doping is mixed. Many scientists regard the genetic modification of athletes as nonsense and completely lacking scientific credibility. In 2001, at a seminar on 'genes in sport' at University College London, renowned biologist Steve Jones likened gene-doping as 'the same ballpark as the babbling nonsense talked about a baldness cure based on gene therapy'.[2] There are good reasons to support such scepticism, given the limited success of gene transfer technology over the last 30 years. If these scientists are correct, then it is easy to sympathise with concerns that serious ethical discussion of these matters is not possible to justify. Indeed, one of the criticisms raised about the present United States President's Council on Bioethics is precisely of this nature. (Turner 2003) In a world where there exist far more real harms and suffering which could be alleviated by medical technology, research and policy, to discuss something so trivial as genetically modified athletes, seems misguided.

Yet there are good reasons to suppose that the application of some scientific studies can have implications for identifying 'performance genes' or finding ways of modifying human performance in sport. Indeed, it is the potentially unsafe use of this technology that gives rise to the ethical concern in the sports world. There is a fear that athletes will try to genetically modify themselves and, in the process, significantly harm themselves. Indeed, many of the supporters of anti-doping have a serious concern that it leads to athletes killing themselves, as was most visibly shown by the death of Tommy Simpson in 1967 during the Tour de France. Currently, research implicated for gene doping includes modifications to growth factors such as IGF-1 (Lamsam et al. 1997; Barton-Davis et al. 1998; Martinek et al. 2000; Goldspink 2001), PGC-1alpha (Lin et al. 2002), recombinant EPO (Svensson et al. 1997) and the ACE gene (Gayagay et al. 1998; Montgomery et al. 1998; Montgomery et al. 1999; Brull et al. 2001). In addition to these methods of modification, scientists are also working towards identifying performance genes which, while not requiring any bodily manipulation, might allow talent scouts to identify who will be the next generation of elite athletes by examining a genetic profile (Rankinen et al. 2006). Indeed, being able to utilise genetic screening is seen also as a way of ensuring that athletes do not participate in sports that are genetically risky for them, such as is the concern about head trauma in relation to boxing (McCrory 2001).

There are also good reasons to ignore the scepticism surrounding gene-doping or, at least, to recognise that the criticisms of this *imagined ethics* appear to emerge from a view of bioethics based on health-care priorities, which is only part of what matters to the development of informed ethical arguments about medicine. The ethical debate about gene-doping is more than just a discussion about what is ethical in sport and medicine, or how sport can be protected from another illegal form of performance enhancement. It is also about more than the allocation of medical research funding. However, one cannot ignore the lure of anti-doping research funds for genetic scientists, some of whom might rely on such funds to pursue their research into genetics. Indeed, the apparent interest of such scientists in sport might actually be little more than scientists trying to gain funding for research they see has value outside sport entirely, as might be said of work concerned with growth factors. The ethics of gene-doping is about further questioning what it is that is threatened by new technology. Sport offers a rich, human and social context where what matters most is placed into question and it is not entirely unfamiliar to bioethicists.

Sport and Bioethics: A Familiar Past

In the 1990s, sport was a key agenda item in the Hastings Center's project on the 'Prospect of Technologies Aimed at the Enhancement of Human Capacities', which gave rise to the volume edited by Eric Parens (1998). In this text, frequent references to sport help to elucidate what it is about enhancement that people find so alarming. Discussions describe how enhancement appears to undermine human excellence, the intrinsic value of our practices, or the means-end progression from novice to expert (Brock 1998; Cole-Turner 1998) In so doing, enhancement is described as 'cheating' the activity, or undermining its value, even contributing to human suffering by leaving our cultural pursuits more impoverished (McKenny 1998). On such a view, sport is characterised as having value partly because of the *chance factor* or, as Parens describes it, 'fragility', which this is threatened by enhancement technologies (Parens 1995).

A number of these issues have been raised elsewhere in literature on philosophy of sport, where, since the 1980s, arguments have been made about the problem with doping (Brown 1980; Hoberman 1992). Indeed, the problem of doping has featured in the Hastings Center Report before. In 1983, Thomas Murray described the 'coercive power of drugs in sport', arguing that 'the use of performance enhancing drugs is ethically undesirable because it is coercive, has significant potential for harm, and advances no social value' (Murray 1983, 30). This was followed shortly by another Hastings collaborative publication, which included a chapter on drugs and sport ethics (Murray 1984). Soon after, Norman Fost developed his 'sceptical view' on banning drugs from sport (Fost 1986). Sport has also been used to question the limits of health and to argue in favour of understanding health as a socially constructed idea, to the extent that the pursuit of health as a justification for using genetic technology is misleading (Sade 1995; Boyd 2000). In contrast, Chadwick uses sport as a basis for questioning the limits of health care, asking whether athletes who take greater risks with their health should be entitled to the same level of care as low risk-takers (Chadwick 1987).

Sport is also used in bioethics as a paradigmatic example of unethical practice for medical therapy, where, for example, genetic modification in sport would not be acceptable, since sport is too trivial an activity to require the use of such important and expensive technology (Glover 1984). Glover even uses sport as a hypothetical test case for what the future might look like where genetically modified athletes are the norm. He argues that such modifications would lead to sameness and make sport uninteresting, since sport is the kind of activity that relies on creating differences. Ledley uses sport as an unethical example of genetic modification, arguing that it would not satisfy Rawls's conditions of fairness by furthering 'inequalities in opportunity without a tangible prospect of benefiting those who remain at a disadvantage of furthering a state of equal basic liberties' (Ledley 1994, 161). Similarly, Little argues that sport is a useful case to explain the limits of fairness. She argues that it is unreasonable to expect fairness in sport and, for this reason, unfairness in genetic capacity is not a basis for utilising technology that might correct this inequality (Little 1998).

There is a lot to argue with in these uses of sport as an example to support bioethical conclusions. For example, sport is often used to portray a dystopian future, where genetically modified athletes are imagined as inhuman or superhuman and where this has resulted from maniacal parents hell-bent on making sure their children succeed. Indeed, one might account for the considerable press coverage that genetically modified athletes has created on this basis. In contrast, sport is also often used as a basis for justifying enhancement technology, as if genetic modification is just another way that people can go about improving health and prospects, like placing our children into sports clubs (Soderberg 1998).

With the exception of Tamburrini and Tännsjö's anthology (Tamburrini and Tännsjö 2005), it is intriguing that this use of sport in bioethics has emerged almost without recourse to literature within the philosophy of sport, which, since 1972, when Paul Weiss founded the Philosophic Society for the Study of Sport (now the International Association for the Philosophy of Sport), has been debating the ethics of performance. Literature has challenged whether doping really undermines the means-end distinction and even questioned whether this matters, since there are many other examples of legal performance-modifiers that have a similar effect but which do not cause alarm. Sport ethicists have also challenged the concepts of 'cheating' and 'fair play', arguing that sport provides unique examples where these ideas do not fit with traditional interpretations (Simon 1991; Loland 2002). Even Parens's concern (Parens 1995) for the value of fragility and chance appear in Bailey (1980), when debating what conditions are worth controlling within the sporting contest to ensure fairness but to preserve spontaneity and surprise.

Despite this lack of conversation between these two areas of philosophical enquiry, there are important overlaps between what each has written, as these examples suggest. Further support can be found in Juengst's articulation of intrinsic value in sport (Juengst 1998), which is complemented by Morgan's application of MacIntyrean articulations of sport ethics (MacIntyre 1985; Morgan 1994), where the practice of sport is defined by the distinction between internal and external goods. Where technology seems to undermine the internal goods by collapsing the distinction between the novice and the expert, this is when sports must re-consider the value of the innovation, though this can comprise innovation in technology as well as rules. However, clearly not all examples of technological innovation have this effect on sports.

Gene-doping

In 2003, the World Anti-Doping Agency included a prohibition of gene doping in sport within its international anti-doping code, which reads as follows:

> II. PROHIBITED METHODS....
> C. GENE DOPING
> Gene or cell doping is defined as the non-therapeutic use of genes, genetic elements and/or cells that have the capacity to enhance athletic performance. (World Anti-Doping Agency 2003)

The kind of arguments used to justify this reaction is not complicated to review. While the WADA code makes reference to the 'spirit of sport' that is threatened by doping, the overwhelming concern about doping remains that the use of an experimental science such as gene transfer would be significantly dangerous and medical malpractice partly for this reason. It would also be performance-enhancing, which means that two of the three criteria within the WADA code are already engaged, even before considering the moral concerns. As such, policy relies on a straightforward medical-ethical model, where therapeutic applications of medicine are acceptable and enhancement or non-therapeutic applications are not. On this basis, it might suffice to respond by utilising Juengst's criticism of applying the medical model to inappropriate contexts, such as sport (Juengst 1998), and to argue that sport should not be subject to similar standards. Yet, further criticisms can be made on the basis of how this discussion has evolved.

Very little debate has taken place about gene-doping within the sporting world outside WADA. Indeed, in 2003, when WADA distributed copies of its 2004 anti-doping code, it became very clear how sport policy debate takes place on a more local level. Before that time, no sports federation mentioned anything about gene-doping and yet, once the draft was available, it was possible to find references to it almost immediately in the websites of sports federations. There is, I suggest, no critical ethical community within sports federations that informs this conversation. Indeed, I would argue that WADA begets such a situation, as its hard-line policy of 'comply, or you can't play' applies to all federations who hope to participate in international competition, driven largely by an interest to maintain Olympic sport status.

It is important to remember that WADA emerged out of the International Olympic Committee and has been chaired from its inception by Richard W. Pound, estranged (and re-embraced) executive of the IOC who, among other things, was largely responsible for making the Olympics a financially viable entity through his negotiation of broadcasting rights during the Samaranch reign. Indeed, the establishment of WADA emerged partly out of a crisis with the IOC credibility and, perhaps more importantly, after the 1998 scandals of the Tour de France where the culture of doping was made so visible and endemic. The criticism of the medical model of ethics in sport can be seen as a broader limitation of anti-doping, which emerged in the post-war climate of medical ethics. The beginning of anti-doping, with the establishment of the IOC Medical Commission in the 1960s, gives some indication of the kinds of values that would underpin the ethics of performance enhancement in elite sport.

These various circumstances have limited how the ethics of performance enhancement have been formulated and, specifically, how gene doping is theorised within anti-doping policy. A number of reactions to this can be made. First, it can be contested that the medical model of ethics is not appropriate to apply to sport, as articulated by Juengst (1998). On this basis, Juengst argues that the ethical concerns specific to practices cannot be applied in a top-down fashion. One sporting example of how this might arise entails the relationship between the athlete and the physician, whose relationship might be regarded as different from a standard patient-doctor relationship. Very often, the athlete's physician has an interest in making the athlete well for competition, rather than simply well. Indeed, medicine is often used in sport to diminish pain sensations to permit an athlete to play through injury. While this might be considered questionable on the standard medical model, the appropriateness of this model might not apply here.

Second, the so-called ethical community within sport that is in need of protection by anti-doping policy makers is largely imagined, and it is unreasonable to assume that there is a clear ethical voice about performance modification. Indeed, a lesser-known attempt to provide such a voice was the OATH initiative – Olympic Athletes Together Honourably. Now seeming to have disappeared entirely from history, OATH comprised a diverse range of people – academics, scientists, athletes – who set about creating a lengthy manifesto on sport ethics. Despite its being presented to the IOC in 2001, OATH disappeared due to lack of funding. One might argue that if such a voice cannot receive the support it deserves, then it cannot be assumed that there is a clear commitment to democratise sport ethics. To further support this claim about an imagined ethical community, one might pose a case that tests this singular voice. For example, what should be the ethical stance taken on something like hypobaric (altitude) chambers (Baker and Hopkins 1998; Levine 2006) or the FastSkin swimming suit from Sydney 2000 (Magdalinski 2000), each of which also enhance performance? For these examples, and many others like them, the presumed ethical conclusions are far less straightforward and, if genetic modification were able to avoid the doping-like rhetoric, it might be regarded with similar ambiguity. Indeed, the tendency to frame gene-doping as just another form of doping has jeopardised the debate about its value considerably.

A third criticism of how gene-doping has been theorised so far concerns the broader implications of genetics. The successfulness of policy on gene-doping must acknowledge the broader bioethical ramifications of genetics. If one contrasts the development of the gene-doping debate with the discussion about drug use in sport, obvious discrepancies appear. Whereas it is possible to claim that anti-doping policy has been of critical importance to governmental debates about drug abuse, no such links appear with regard to gene-doping. Indeed, the (potentially problematic) example of the US President's Council on Bioethics does not find gene doping to be obviously unethical at all (US President's Council on Bioethics 2002a). Rather, its use might be seen as consistent with an *ethics of technologisation* in sport, which appears to reflect current values in elite sport. In contrast, with regard to anti-doping more broadly, WADA has long-established links with governments of Olympic nations, as well as institutions such as the European Union and the United Nations in its 'fight' against doping. Yet, in relation to gene-doping, WADA does not appear to be in dialogue with bioethical committees, legal authorities, think-tanks or governmental advisory boards. In this sense, policy-making concerning gene-doping has the potential to be inconsistent with broader bioethical and bio-legal decisions concerning acceptability. Indeed, the legal disparities between sporting authorities and wider social obligations to athletes' rights is precisely what is discussed by the ALRC (Australia Law Reform Commission 2003). Recognising this broader context is crucial for sports authorities and should not permit them to implement a fixed policy on the role of genetics in sport performance.

A final response to the debate on gene-doping is related to my previous claim, though it relies significantly on conjecture. If it is reasonable to imagine that gene transfer technology will play a greater role in society in the future, then it is unreasonable for anti-doping policy to rely on essentialising human performance in the way that it currently does. Thus, the ethics of sport based on some notion of 'natural' performance becomes increasingly difficult to sustain as more diverse kinds of human arise from the use of medical technology. While claims about a natural human do not feature quite so clearly in anti-doping discussions any more, an appeal to 'God-given talents' remains critical to how anti-doping is justified. Admittedly, this is partly why there is such concern about genetic modification; because it challenges this naturalness. Yet, this ethical view of sport performances appears unsustainable in an age where various reproductive technologies disrupt the notion of the natural considerably. This need not be seen as an affront to anti-doping policy, indeed, quite the contrary. It can provide a basis for recognising why many kinds of performance enhancement do not challenge the value of sport performance at all. Genetically modified athletes will still need to train hard to be elite and it would be no short cut to an elite performance. While this defence also applies to the drug-use case, genetic modification does not have the anti-social baggage that drugs have. As such, it would be premature to dismiss its value as a life-enhancing or, more accurately, health-enhancing innovation for society and sports.

Clearly, there are further ethical arguments that must be considered in a response to gene-doping, which I have not addressed here. I have not yet mentioned the challenge to 'fair play' that gene doping might yield. As well, I have not mentioned ethical concerns about the coercive and potentially divisive consequence of accepting genetically modified athletes into competition. Yet, with the social force that anti-doping has, it is no small task to suggest that its ethical basis might need revisiting. However, I would suggest that my proposal for reform is modest and should not be construed as an 'anything goes' argument. Rather, a straightforward dismissal of gene-doping, as is taking place in current sport policy, is not sufficient and will encounter difficulties for the reasons I have outlined.

Beyond these arguments, there are still gaps in the ethical discourse concerning gene-doping. For example, no prohibition or statement has been made about the ethics of using genetic information to select elite athletes. Thus, investment into identifying performance genes, which might be correlated with elite performance capacities, is not considered to be a prohibited use of the technology. This is interesting, since precisely this application is criticised by the Australian Law Reform Commission, which argues that it could seriously compromise the legal status of the athlete (Australia Law Reform Commission 2003). In its report, the ALRC questions whether sports authorities would be legally permitted to request such information. Also, the WADA position derives from a concern about somatic-cell modification and the use of pharmacogenomics, which might yield 'wonder-drugs' that are undetectable. It is not directed to the prospect of germ-line cell modification. While the scientific reaction might be that there is no need to consider this prospect yet, it has already been identified that WADA is not aiming to develop policy based on present-day applications of genetic technology. Rather, it is supposed to be about the business of developing a robust ethical policy for gene transfer technology. For this reason, the ethical status of genetically modified embryos might be worth considering, particularly since the unsustainability of a prohibition on such athletes further reveals the weakness of the current strategy. In short, it is not acceptable to prohibit genetically modified humans from participating in sport, just because they were born that way.

Conclusion

In part, the reasons for wanting to defend gene-doping emerge out of my concern for the methodological limitations of anti-doping and the desire to see anti-doping embrace a broader bioethical debate about genetics, the ethics of enhancement and the use of medicine in sport more generally. The kinds of arguments that have emerged in the last 40 years of bioethical discussion have not informed the ethical discussion about doping in sport very much at all, which seems very unfortunate. Within academic ethical debates, neither have links been made to critical developments in bioethics. For example, despite numerous allusions to the importance of establishing the value of 'humanness' as a basis for what makes sport special, there have been nearly no references to bioethical discussions about humanness, dignity or personhood. This is not to say that anti-doping has been critically informed by academic debates in the philosophy of sport either. Far from it. Part of the explanation for this is historical, though much more of it would appear to be institutional. Sport philosophers have rarely published in medical journals and scientists concerned about ethics have rarely engaged with (and are often dismissive of) sport ethics or bioethics. Yet sport offers a particularly rich context where one can develop an ethical critique of genetic technology (Miah 2004; Tamburrini and Tännsjö 2005). In this sense, philosophy of sport offers something useful to the development of bioethics, as the references to it suggest. For one thing, the global context of sport raises challenging philosophical issues about the universality of moral principles – are sport ethics universal? In a world that remains befuddled by the human cloning debate and the internationality of ethics related to human genetics, WADA is bypassing that confusion and asserting what is right and proper for humans by prohibiting gene-doping on the basis of a contested assumption that there are unified codes of ethics in sport.

The prospect of gene-doping can make it impossible to avoid making these connections between bioethics and sport ethics. Inevitably, any policy concerning the use of genetic technology in sport will find itself beholden to broader bioethical policies about the use of gene transfer technology. For example, in a world that permits the use of gene transfer technology for therapeutic purposes, it would be inconceivable that sports authorities could prohibit such athletes from competition, just because they were genetically modified. In this respect, gene-doping is unlike any other method of performance enhancement in sport. Moreover, the world of sport is reacting to gene-doping in a way that is unparalleled by any other form of doping. For once, it has an opportunity to derive ethical guidelines before the technology is realised, a problem that has inhibited much of its strategy for other methods of doping. Yet, there are good reasons for avoiding the straightforward classification of genetic modification as any other form of doping, which I have tried to outline here.

None of the discussions about gene doping have even considered the debates taking place in the AAAS, the ALRC or the US President's Council. Yet, each of these organisations presents quite different accounts of the critical ethical issues arising from gene technology in sport. If the WADA prohibition can be seen as a precautionary statement, then this need not be a lost opportunity to use gene-doping as a means to re-evaluating what matters in sport, bearing in mind that it might have changed since anti-doping began. However, the ethical debate about gene-doping must take place on a far wider scale, and anti-doping policy-makers must be prepared to accept that it might be a far better strategy to seek ways of legitimising such methods of performance enhancement rather than ban them. The genetically modified athlete is not somebody who can straightforwardly be labelled as a 'cheat' and this is critical to realise when beginning to discuss the ethical implications of this technology. After all, genetically modified athletes might not have altered themselves at all, but might have been brought about by the *knowledge* provided by genetics. Alternatively, if we are discussing whether a genetically modified athlete should be allowed to compete or not, it is important to recognise that the discussion might involve the offspring of genetically modified humans. As such, we would only indirectly consider such persons to be genetically modified and the extent to which they could be labelled cheats becomes far more complex, even if they have a competitive advantage in sport.

These concerns are consistent with a further criticism of anti-doping that, predominantly, it continues to penalise the athlete in the 'culture of doping' as described by Lord Charles Dubin in his post-Ben Johnson report (Dubin 1990). Dubin's conclusions were significant for identifying that it is not just the athlete who creates the doping culture of sport. Rather, it is a range of people and professions that make it possible. Houlihan (1999; 2004) has written extensively on the weaknesses of solely targeting and punishing athletes, stressing the importance of education and sanctions for people within the athlete's entourage, including team physicians. Yet, athletes remain the target for criticism when doping cases arises. One of the most recent examples of this was tennis player Greg Rusedski's positive test for nandrolone, which illustrates the inadequacies of the 'anti-athlete' approach to doping. While there was no question about whether the results were reliable, it transpired that the consumption of the substance arose from a nutritional supplement, which was distributed by the Association of Tennis Professionals. Rusedski could not be held responsible for having tested positive. The Rusedski case provided unequivocal evidence that the very standards required of athletes by sports authorities to ensure they do not consume prohibited substances are not met by the institutions themselves who set them. As such, the moral high ground so often taken against the 'guilty' athlete overlooks the more detailed and complex circumstances within which positive tests arise and the conceptual difficulties with establishing what constitutes an ethically permissible method of performance enhancement in sport.

NOTES

1. See www.genedoping.com
2. D. Powell, 'Spectre of gene doping raises its head as athletes see possibilities', *The Times* (London), 29 November 2001.

REFERENCES

AAAS (AMERICAN ASSOCIATION FOR THE ADVANCEMENT OF SCIENCE). 2003. Bigger, faster, stronger: Genetic enhancement and athletics. Symposium at annual meeting, 18 Feb., Denver, CO. Available at http://health.ucsd.edu/news/2003/02_18_Friedmann.html, accessed 7 June 2007.

AUSTRALIA LAW REFORM COMMISSION. 2001. Protection of human genetic information – 12. Other services and contexts. Issues paper 26, available at http://www.austlii.edu.au/au/other/alrc/publications/issues/26/, accessed 7 June 2007.

———. 2003. *ALRC 96: Essentially Yours.* Sydney: Australian Law Reform Commission of the Australian National Government.

BAILEY, C.I. 1980. Sport and the element of chance. *Journal of Sport Behaviour* 3 (2): 69 – 75.

BAKER, A. and W.G. HOPKINS. 1998. Altitude training for sea-level competition. *Sportscience: Training & Technology. Internet Society for Sport Science*, available at http://sportsci.org/traintech/altitude/wgh.html, accessed 7 June 2007.

BARTON-DAVIS, E.R., D.I. SHOTURMA, A. MUSARO, N. ROSENTHAL and H.L. SWEENEY. 1998. Viral mediated expression of insulin-like growth factor I blocks the aging-related loss of skeletal muscle function. *Proceedings of the National Academy of Sciences* (USA) 95: 15603 – 7.

BOYD, K.M. 2000. Disease, illness, sickness, health, healing and wholeness: Exploring some elusive concepts. *Journal of Medical Ethics: Medical Humanities* 26 (1): 9 – 17.

BROCK, D.W. 1998. Enhancements of human function: Some distinctions for policymakers. In *Enhancing Human Traits: Ethical and Social Implications*, edited by E. Parens. Washington, DC: Georgetown University Press: 48 – 69.

BROWN, W.M. 1980. Ethics, drugs and sport. *Journal of the Philosophy of Sport* VII: 15 – 23.

BRULL, D., S. DHAMRAIT, S. MYERSON, J. ERDMANN, V. REGITZ-ZAGROSEK, M. WORLD, D. PENNELL, S.E. HUMPRHIES and H. MONTGOMERY. 2001. Bradykinin B2bkr receptor polymorphism and left-ventricular growth response. *The Lancet* 358 (6 Oct.): 1155 – 6.

CHADWICK, R.F. 1987. Having children: Introduction. In *Ethics, Reproduction and Genetic Control*, edited by R.F. Chadwick. London: Routledge: 3 – 43.

COLE-RURNER, R. 1998. Do means matter? In *Enhancing Human Traits: Ethical and Social Implications*, edited by E. Parens. Washington, DC: Georgetown University Press: 151 – 61.

DUBIN, C.L. 1990. *Commission of Inquiry into the Use of Drugs and Banned Practices Intended to Increase Athletic Performance.* Ottawa: Canadian Government Publishing Centre.

FOST, N. 1986. Banning drugs in sports: A skeptical view. *Hastings Center Report* 16: 5 – 10.

GAYAGAY, GEORGE., BING. YU, BRETT. HAMBLY, TANYA. BOSTON, ALAN. HAHN, DAVID S. CELERMAJER and R. J. TRENT. 1998. Elite endurance athletes and the Ace I Allele – the role of genes in athletic performance. *Human Genetics* 103 (1): 48 – 50.

GLOVER, J. 1984. *What Sort of People Should There Be?* Harmondsworth: Penguin.

GOLDSPINK, G. 2001. Gene expression in skeletal muscle. *Biochemical Society Transactions* 30: 285 – 90.

HOBERMAN, J.M. 1992. *Mortal Engines: The Science of Performance and the Dehumanization of Sport.* New York: The Free Press (reprinted 2001, The Blackburn Press).

HOULIHAN, B. 1999. *Dying to Win: Doping in Sport and the Development of Anti-Doping Policy.* Strasburg: Council of Europe Publishing.

————. 2004. Civil rights, doping control and the world anti-doping code. *Sport in Society* 7 (3): 420 – 37.

INTERNATIONAL OLYMPIC COMMITTEE. 2001. IOC Gene Therapy Working Group – Conclusion. Press release, International Olympic Committee, Lausanne, available at http://www.olympic. org/uk/news/publications/press_uk.asp?release=179, accessed 7 June 2007.

JUENGST, E.T. 1998. What does enhancement mean? In *Enhancing Human Traits: Ethical and Social Implications*, edited by E. Parens. Washington, DC: Georgetown University Press: 29 – 47.

KANE, D. 2004. Athletics, genetic enhancement and ethics. American Association for the Advancement of Science press release, available at http://www.aaas.org/news/releases/ 2004/0224athalete.shtml, accessed 7 June 2007.

LAMSAM, C., F.H. FU, P.D. ROBBINS and C.H. EVANS. 1997. Gene therapy in sports medicine. *Sports Medicine* 25 (2): 73 – 7.

LEDLEY, F.D. 1994. Distinguishing genetics and eugenics on the basis of fairness. *Journal of Medical Ethics* 20: 157 – 64.

LEE, S., E.R. BARTON, H.L. SWEENEY and R.P. FARRAR. 2004. Viral expression of insulin-like growth factor-I enhances muscle hypertrophy in resistance-trained rats. *Journal of Applied Physiology* 96: 1097 – 1104.

LEVINE, B.D. 2006. Editorial: should 'artificial' high altitude environments be considered doping? *Scandinavian Journal of Medicine and Science in Sports* 16: 297 – 301.

LIN, J., H. WU, P.T. TARR, C. ZHANG, Z. WU, O. BOSS, L.F. MICHAEL, P. PUIGSERVER, E. ISOTANI, E.N. OLSON, B.B. LOWELL, R. BASSEL-DUBY and B.M. SPIEGELMANN. 2002. Transcriptional co-activator Pgc-1 drives the formation of slow-twitch muscle fibres. *Nature* 418: 797 – 801.

LITTLE, M.O. 1998. Cosmetic surgery, suspect norms, and the ethics of complicity. In *Enhancing Human Traits: Ethical and Social Implications*, edited by E. Parens. Washington, DC: Georgetown University Press: 162 – 76.

LOLAND, S. 2002. *Fair Play in Sport: A Moral Norm System*. London and New York: Routledge.

MACINTYRE, A. 1985. *After Virtue: A Study in Moral Theory*. 2nd edn. London: Duckworth.

MCCRORY, P. 2001. Ethics, molecular biology, and sports medicine. *British Journal of Sports Medicine* 35 (3): 142 – 3.

MCKENNY, G.P. 1998. Enhancements and the ethical significance of vulnerability. In *Enhancing Human Traits: Ethical and Social Implications*, edited by E. Parens. Washington, DC: Georgetown University Press: 222 – 37.

MAGDALINSKI, T. 2000. Performance technologies: Drugs and Fastskin at the Sydney 2000 Olympics. *Media International Australia* 97 (Nov.): 59 – 69.

MARTINEK, V., F.H. FU and J. HUARD. 2000. Gene therapy and tissue engineering in sports medicine. *The Physician and Sports Medicine* 28 (2), available at http://www.physsportsmed.com/ issues/2000/02_00/huard.htm, accessed 7 June 2007.

MIAH, A. 2004. *Genetically Modified Athletes: Biomedical Ethics, Gene Doping and Sport*. London and New York: Routledge.

MONTGOMERY, H., R. MARSHALL, H. HEMINGWAY, S. MYERSON, P. CLARKSON, C. DOLLERY, M. HAYWARD, D.E. HOLLIMAN, M. JUBB, M. WORLD, E.L. THOMAS, A.E. BRYNES, N. SAEED, M. BARNARD, J.D. BELL, K. PRASAD, M. RAYSON, P.J. TALMUD and S.E. HUMPHRIES. 1998. Human gene for physical performance. *Nature* 393 (21): 221 – 2.

MONTGOMERY, H., P. CLARKSON, M. BARNARD, J. BELL, A. BRYNES, C. DOLLERY, J. HAJNAL, H. HEMINGWAY, D. MERCER, P. JARMAN, R. MARSHALL, K. PRASAD, M. RAYSON, N. SAEED, P. TALMUD, L. THOMAS, M. JUBB, M. WORLD and S. HUMPHRIES. 1999. Angiotensin-converting-enzyme gene insertion/ deletion polymorphism and response to physical training. *The Lancet* 353 (13): 541 – 5.

MORGAN, W.J. 1994. *Leftist Theories of Sport: A Critique and Reconstruction*. Urbana, IL: University of Illinois Press.

MURRAY, T.H. 1983. The coercive power of drugs in sports. *Hastings Center Report* (August): 24 – 30.

———. 1984. Drugs, sports, and ethics. In *Feeling Good and Doing Better*, edited by T.H. Murray, W. Gaylin and R. Macklin. Clifton, NJ: Humana Press: 107 – 26.

PARENS, E. 1995. The goodness of fragility: On the prospect of genetic technologies aimed at the enhancement of human capacities. *Kennedy Institute of Ethics Journal* 5 (2): 141 – 53.

———, ed. 1998. *Enhancing Human Traits: Ethical and Social Implications*. Washington, DC: Georgetown University Press.

RANKINEN, T., M.S. BRAY, J.M. HAGBERG, L. PÉRUSSE, S.M. ROTH, B. WOLFARTH and C. BOUCHARD. 2006. The human gene map for performance and health-related fitness phenotypes: The 2005 update. *Medicine and Science in Sport & Exercise* 38 (11): 1863 – 88.

SADE, R.M. 1995. A theory of health and disease: The objectivist-subjectivist dichotomy. *Journal of Medicine and Philosophy* 20 (5): 513 – 25.

SIMON, R.L. 1991. *Fair Play: Sport, Values, and Society*. Boulder, CO: Westview Press.

SODERBERG, W. 1998. Genetic enhancement of a child's memory: A search for a private and public morality. Paper presented at the 20th World Congress of Philosophy, Boston, MA.

SVENSSON, E.C., H.B. BLACK, D.L. DUGGER, S.K. TRIPATHY, E. GOLDWASSER, Z. HAO, L. CHU and J.M. LEIDEN. 1997. Long-term erythropoietin expression in rodents and non-human primates following intramuscular injection of a replication-defective adenoviral vector. *Human Gene Therapy* 8 (15): 1797 – 1806.

TAMBURRINI, C. and T. TÄNNSJÖ, eds. 2005. *Genetic Technology and Sport: Ethical Questions, Ethics and Sport*. Abingdon and New York: Routledge.

TURNER, L. 2003. Has the President's Council on Bioethics missed the boat? *British Medical Journal* 327: 629.

US PRESIDENT'S COUNCIL ON BIOETHICS. 2002a. *Session 4: Enhancement 2: Potential for Genetic Enhancements in Sports*. Washington, DC: The President's Council on Bioethics (available at http://www.bioethics.gov/transcripts/jul02/session4.html, accessed 7 June 2007).

———. 2002b. *Sixth Meeting: Session 7: Enhancement 5: Genetic Enhancement of Muscle*. Washington, DC: The President's Council on Bioethics (available at http://www.bioethics.gov/transcripts/sep02/session7.html, accessed 7 June 2007).

WORLD ANTI-DOPING AGENCY. 2002. WADA conference sheds light on the potential of gene doping. Press release, World Anti-Doping Agency, New York, available at http://www.wada-ama.org, accessed 7 June 2007.

———. 2003. International standard for the prohibited list 2004. Available at http://www.wada-ama.org/docs/web/standards_harmonization/code/list_standard_2004.pdf, accessed 7 June 2007.

———. 2005. *The Stockholm Declaration*. Montreal: World Anti-Doping Agency.

RESPECTING PRIVACY IN DETECTING ILLEGITIMATE ENHANCEMENTS IN ATHLETES

Sarah Teetzel

This paper explores the degree of privacy athletes can expect and demand in the era of genetic technology in sport. Detecting genetic enhancements in sport, and consequently doping violations, using genetic tests is problematic because testing requires access to athletes' genetic information, and accessing genetic information creates many potential privacy issues and concerns throughout the world. Whether it is morally acceptable to subject athletes to the tests used to detect genetic modifications in sport is taken up in this paper, and I argue that the elite sport movement faces an ethical dilemma since rules prohibit athletes from utilising certain substances, methods and procedures, but the testing methods needed to ensure compliance with the rules are controversial and at odds with a reasonable expectation of privacy.

Resumen

Este artículo explora el grado de intimidad que los atletas pueden esperar y exigir en la era de la tecnología genética en el deporte. La detección de mejoras genéticas en el deporte, y consecuentemente de violaciones por dopaje, usando análisis genéticos es problemática porque tales pruebas requieren acceso a la información genética de los atletas, y el acceder a la información genética crea potencialmente muchos problemas y preocupaciones por todo el mundo que atañen a la intimidad. Este artículo considera si es moralmente aceptable el obligar a los atletas a someterse a los análisis utilizados para detectar modificaciones genéticas en el deporte, y discute que el deporte de élite encara un dilema, ya que las reglas prohíben a los atletas la utilización de ciertas sustancias, métodos, y procedimientos, mas los métodos de análisis que se requieren para asegurar conformidad con las reglas son polémicos y están en desacuerdo con una expectativa razonable de intimidad.

Zusammenfassung

Dieser Artikel befasst sich mit dem den Athleten zustehenden Grad an Privatheit in Bezug auf Sport im Zeitalter der Gentechnik. Die Suche nach genetischen Maßnahmen zur Leistungssteigerung im Sport und die damit verbundenen Verletzungen der Anti-Dopingrichtlinien machen konsequenterweise Gen-Dopingtests erforderlich. Die Verwendung solcher Tests ist aber nicht unproblematisch, da sie einen Einblick in die genetischen Informationen der Athleten erfordern.

Der Zugriff auf solcherlei Daten wäre weltweit von einer Vielzahl von Problemen und Bedenken begleitet. Ob es moralisch vertretbar ist, derartige Tests bei Sportlern durchzuführen um genetischen Veränderzungen auf die Spur zu kommen, ist Gegenstand dieses Aufsatzes. Ich behaupte, dass sich der Leistungssport seit dem Verbot der Verwendung bestimmter Substanzen, Methoden und Verfahren einem ethischen Dilemma ausgesetzt sieht, denn die Testverfahren zur Sicherstellung des regelgerechten Wettbewerbs sind umstritten und sie stehen im Konflikt mit einer vernünftigen Wahrung der Privatsphäre.

摘要

本文旨在探討運動界中的基因科技時代中，有關運動員的隱私可期待與要求的程度。偵查出運動中的運用基因提高表現的情況，而導致禁藥的違法使用，使用基因檢測等存在著許多問題，因為檢測需要使用到運動員的基因背景資料，如此便引發出許多潛在的私人議題與關心。本文從事的研究即是檢測運動員使用基因修改的現象，道德上是否可以接受。我認為頂尖運動的發展遇到了一個倫理課題上的二難，因為規則上禁止運動員使用特殊的違法物質、方法和手續，但是檢測方法卻又必須擔保符合規則，如此是有爭議的，並且和合理的隱私期待不一致。

Respecting Privacy in Detecting Illegitimate Enhancements in Athletes

Privacy is a complicated notion in sport. Medal winners and athletes drawn at random can expect to have their urine and blood tested at all major athletic competitions as well as throughout the year in out-of-competition tests. When national and international anti-doping agencies decide to test an athlete for the use of performance-enhancing substances or methods, the athlete must declare his or her whereabouts, submit to the testing and provide the requested blood or urine sample under observation; to do otherwise is taken as an admission of guilt and a 'positive' test result for doping. Privacy advocates might maintain that this system does not respect the privacy that athletes, as human beings, are entitled to receive, but this claim is contestable. Consequently, a recurring theme in the philosophical literature on privacy is the uncertainty regarding how much privacy a person ought to be able to expect and demand.[1]

How much privacy an athlete can expect in the sporting world is even more unclear due to the prerequisite conditions sport-governing organisations require athletes to adhere to in order to participate. At first glance, participation in elite sport appears to be an instance where a person's expectations of privacy are threatened by rules imposed by an outside body. The challenges to privacy that athletes face as a result of drug testing programmes in sport create an interesting case study to analyse the different societal expectations placed on athletes in their roles as elite athletes compared to their entitlements as members of the human race.[2] This paper explores the degree of privacy an athlete living in a free and democratic society can reasonably expect and demand in the era of genetic enhancements, gene-doping and illicit uses of genetic technology in sport. A ban on gene-doping in sport requires enforcement through testing, and tests currently used to detect gene-doping provide not only evidence of gene-transfer procedures but also access to the individual's genetic information. Whether it is ethical to subject athletes to the tests used to detect gene-doping in sport is debatable because of the corresponding infringement on the athletes' right to privacy and autonomy that these procedures might entail.

Schneider and Butcher (2001) as well as Thompson (1995) have addressed the ethical issues associated with drug testing in sport, while Munthe (2005) has described the issues arising from the prospect of performing genetic tests on healthy athletes for doping detection purposes. With these issues in mind, the conflict inherent in simultaneously testing for genetic technologies and respecting privacy becomes apparent. The resulting problem can be condensed to four simple, yet contentious, statements: (1) individuals are entitled to expect a certain degree of privacy; (2) athletes are prohibited from undergoing enhancements deemed illegitimate in sport; (3) tests are needed to ensure anti-doping rules are followed; and (4) current tests to detect illegitimate genetic enhancements violate athletes' justifiable expectations of privacy. Thus, the elite sport movement faces an ethical dilemma since rules prohibit athletes from utilising certain substances, methods and procedures, but the testing methods needed to ensure compliance with the rules are controversial and at odds with a reasonable expectation of privacy.

Expectations of Privacy

Privacy issues have been discussed in the law and ethics literature since Warren and Brandeis (1890, 193) defined privacy as 'the right to be left alone' in the *Harvard Law Review*. Since then, numerous philosophers have attempted to fine-tune the definition to serve a multitude of purposes and determine if privacy is a basic human right that humans are entitled to by virtue of their humanness. Parent (as cited in Moore 2003, 315) defines privacy as 'the condition of not having undocumented personal knowledge about one possessed by others', but others are more stringent or encompassing in their definitions. For example, the account of privacy given by McArthur (2001) hinges on what a reasonable modern person would expect rather than on nostalgic and outdated accounts from the past, and Volkman (2003) sees privacy as concerns derived from our rights to life, liberty and property. Clearly, there are several ways of considering the notion of privacy.[3] The difficulties involved in producing a universally accepted definition of privacy have led many philosophers to declare the search for a precise definition to be futile, and as Alfino and Mayes (2003, 3) illustrate, building on Judith Jarvis Thomson's work, 'perhaps the most striking thing about the right to privacy *today* is that nobody seems to have any very clear idea whether it is a right at all'. Widespread consensus on what privacy means and what it entails is unlikely because individuals' values and worldviews often lead them to different interpretations of the notion (Malcolm 2005).

It has been argued that 'privacy is valuable because it protects what [people] deem important in life, such as the intimate sphere or the conditions for autonomous judgement' (Beckman 2005, 98). The protective nature of privacy is evident if one believes that

> Privacy acts as a shield to protect us in various ways, and its value lies in the freedom and independence it provides for us. Privacy shields us not only from interference and pressures that preclude self-expression and the development of relationships, but also from intrusions and pressures arising from others' access to our persons and the details

about us. Threats of information leaks as well as threats of control over our bodies, our activities, and our power to make our own choices give rise to fears that we are being scrutinized, judged, ridiculed, pressured, coerced, or otherwise taken advantage of by others.... Loss of privacy leaves us vulnerable and threatened. (DeCew 1999, 249)

Without assurances of privacy, conformist traditions and behaviours devoid of critical reflection tend to flourish as individuals experience the vulnerability noted by DeCew. In conjunction with the stance that privacy 'is one of our most cherished rights' (Moore 2003, 215) a strong case emerges for granting all individuals a certain degree of privacy.

How far a right to privacy should extend is currently being debated in the medical ethics literature, and the sporting world could benefit from paying attention to this discourse. Privacy is a frequently discussed topic in the contemporary bioethics literature because of the role it plays in treating people as autonomous beings worthy of respect. For example, Beauchamp and Childress (2001) regard privacy as a moral rule that medical professionals and researchers who work with human subjects must respect. Since drug testing and genetic testing of athletes involve procedures and tests that originated in the medical context, it is important to note the reverence that respect for privacy holds in the bioethics and medical ethics fields.

As well, the bioethics and medical ethics literature establishes a strong link between privacy rights and respecting autonomy. Violating a person's privacy fails to respect the person as an autonomous agent because doing so denies him or her the power to control who has access to privileged information about his/her self and body.[4] When medical tests and procedures can analyse our genes and calculate our probable susceptibility to developing certain diseases and disorders, our genes can be considered a gargantuan source of information about our bodies. The results obtained from genetic tests contain very sensitive information that must be guarded carefully to respect and protect a patient or subject's privacy. Support for these sentiments comes from lines of reasoning that appeal to values, autonomy, the strong personal nature of genetic information and the consequences of results for family members with similar genetic codes (Beckman 2005).

Performing tests to detect genetic enhancements could theoretically provide anti-doping agencies with unlimited access to athletes' genetic information. There are more than 160 genes and phenotypes known to affect fitness and health, and anyone with considerable knowledge of genetics and the right equipment can determine much more than if one is predisposed to being an elite athlete (Wolforth et al. 2005). If there is anything people might feel ownership over and have a right not to have to share with others, it may be the information contained within their genetic codes pertaining to their current and future health, which can be described as their genetic book of life (Schneider 2005). This information extends beyond mere knowledge of one's future health and can facilitate several undesirable consequences, such as 'embarrassment, loss of self-esteem, social stigma, isolation, and psychological distress,... economic loss and discrimination in such areas as employment, child custody, insurance, housing, and immigration status' (DeCew 2004, 5). Therefore, genetic information must be protected.

Legitimate and Illegitimate Uses of Gene Therapies in Sport

Gene transfer experts working in conjunction with the World Anti-Doping Agency (WADA) agree that athletes will soon be able to transfer therapeutic and performance-enhancing genes into their bodies to facilitate superior athletic performance. No longer a speculative assumption or a tale of science fiction, gene-doping, many experts predict, will become a reality before the 2008 Olympics in Beijing (Adam 2001). Preliminary gene therapy research shows promise in producing therapeutic benefits in the cardiovascular, neurological, musculoskeletal and respiratory systems, as well as expediting the healing of damaged bones, cartilage, ligaments and other soft tissues, among other ergogenic effects. Hence many therapeutic gene transfer procedures show signs of causing physiological adaptations similar to those gained through chronic exercise, and are expected to enhance athleticism in addition to producing the therapeutic benefits for which they were created.

For an athlete currently using or contemplating the use of banned performance-enhancing drugs, the astonishing and virtually undetectable results produced in animal models and early stages of clinical trials may seem too good to be true. Several geneticists, scientists and philosophers suggest that athletes will turn to genetic modifications to gain an edge on their competitors and enable their bodies to produce never-before-witnessed feats of strength and speed as soon as the technology is available (Miah 2004; Schneider and Friedmann 2006). If athletes are not tested for the use of particular banned substances, or if no reliable tests are available, only an athlete's sense of fair play prevents him or her from breaking the rules and gaining an advantage over competitors who choose to adhere to the rules. The ban on artificially elevating haemoglobin levels before reliable tests for blood doping and erythropoietin (EPO) were discovered exemplifies this scenario; when it was widely known that anti-doping agencies could not distinguish exogenous red blood cells from endogenous ones, many athletes proceeded to violate the rule because they thought they could get away with doing so (Pascual et al. 2004, 176). Effective tests are thus necessary since doping bans only work if they are both enforceable and enforced.

To rid sport of doping and deter athletes from using banned substances, a rigorous global anti-doping programme is required (Fraser 2004). Testing is currently the primary method of catching violators of the World Anti-Doping Code, not the provision of education about the risks of doping and the values of fair play (Malloy and Zakus 2000). For this reason, WADA's proactive classification of genetic enhancements as banned practices in sport generates the need to identify exogenous genes transferred into the body to detect an athlete's abuse of procedures being developed as gene therapies.

Detecting gene transfers in athletes will constitute a considerable challenge and may not be possible without utilising invasive procedures and equipment that is currently unavailable in standard drug-testing facilities. The majority of methods under investigation by researchers affiliated with WADA are invasive and cause an athlete considerable discomfort because detecting the DNA of artificial and transferred genes requires a sample of the tissue containing the modification. On paper this does not sound that difficult, but in reality detecting genetic enhancements in a sample 'would be like looking for the proverbial needle in the haystack and would be unlikely to garner much enthusiasm from athletes given the invasive nature of the biopsies' (McCrory 2003, 192). However, the physical pain that the removal of a tissue sample for genetic analysis will cause is not the only controversial factor drug-testing agencies need to consider; the violation of athletes' privacy caused by tests used to detect illegitimate gene transfer procedures in sport creates the need for further analysis and discussion.

The World Anti-Doping Code currently classifies genetic enhancements as banned practices in sport and unequivocally prohibits the use of such procedures except for therapeutic purposes. International sports federations must endorse and adhere to the code in order to participate in the Olympic Games and other multi-sport competitions. Sport-governing bodies traditionally have expected athletes to play by their rules or participate elsewhere. WADA director Richard Pound offers his, and ostensibly WADA's, motivation and justification for banning gene doping in sport and working with leading gene therapy researchers to develop tests to detect gene doping:

> [Sport] is governed by rules that, however artificial or arbitrary they may be, are freely accepted by the participants. Why a race is 100 or 200 or 1,500 metres does not really matter. Nor does the weight of a shot...the number of members on a team or specifications regarding equipment. Those are the agreed-upon rules. Period. Sport involves even more freedom of choice than participation in society. If you do not agree with the rules in sport, you are entirely free to opt-out, unlike your ability to opt-out of the legal framework of society. But if you do participate, you must accept the rules.[5]

WADA makes the rules pertaining to doping, and substances or methods it deems to cause any two of the following three outcomes are prohibited: (1) enhanced performance; (2) harm to the athlete; or (3) behaviour contrary to the spirit of sport (World Anti-Doping Agency 2003, 15–16). While these criteria are nebulous and ill-defined, athletes must voluntarily agree to adhere to WADA's decisions regarding banned substances and procedures in order to play.

Testing and Privacy Violations

If WADA decides to utilise genetic tests to uncover genetic modifications in athletes, many safeguards will need to be implemented to protect the privacy of those subjected to the tests. In medical settings, doctors, lab technicians and medical personnel involved in genetic testing are able to use advanced technology to access patients' present and future health information because protection measures are in place to ensure the information they access stays out of the public record. It has been argued that family members, twins, insurance companies and employers might want to know the results of genetic tests (Brockett and Tankersley 1997); however, in sport, it is conceivable that reporters and the segment of the population that treats top athletes as bona fide celebrities would also be interested in any juicy or interesting detail contained in an athlete's genetic code. Risks to privacy are minimised by the fact that those working in the medical field must adhere to codes of ethics and standards of conduct that explicitly prohibit sharing information garnered about a patient's current or future health without the patient's consent. Safeguards are therefore in place in the medical field to protect patients' privacy and preserve their trust.

Organisations operating outside the medical field are not obliged to adhere to the same codes of conduct or behaviours upheld by medical professionals and demanded by medical associations. As a result, an individual's privacy may become jeopardised if genetic tests are used in lax environments (Beckman 2005). Performing genetic tests on tissue samples taken from athletes violates their privacy if the samples are taken without permission and the results are announced to the world without their consent. However, this is neither how testing in sport is carried out now nor how it likely will be done in the future (Thompson 1995). Our widely-accepted rights to privacy prevent others from invading our personal spaces and from taking samples from our bodies without our explicit consent to do so, and this is widely acknowledged in sport. It is expected that drug-testing agencies take, and will continue to take, precautions to avoid unduly subjecting athletes to privacy violations. Nonetheless, what the sports world needs to make clear is who will have access to the results of genetic tests and what they will do with the results. Before adding genetic tests to the drug-testing repertoire, WADA must address this issue and develop appropriate and scrupulous policies to ensure confidentiality will be maintained.

Strategies to safeguard the results of genetic tests are not the only consideration in need of further specification and discussion. Pound's argument that athletes can opt out of participating if they do not agree with the rules is problematic if the testing methods athletes rely on to ensure their competitors comply with the rules contravene acceptable standards of privacy and autonomy, and if the only other option is to not take part. The consent that athletes give to anti-doping agencies to have their blood and urine analysed for traces of prohibited substances is not without coercion in many cases.[6] However, WADA maintains that 'the strict liability criteria and sanctions [it uses] are fair within accepted principles of international law and human rights' (Honour 2004, 144).

Individuals can consent to waive their rights to 'privacy, confidentiality, non-discrimination, and autonomous decision making' if they so choose (Hayray and Takale 2001, 403 – 5). Indeed, it is because of this waiver that WADA can require blood and urine samples from athletes without creating too much controversy, and why many athletes willingly provide the samples. However, the coercive elements that underlie an athlete's agreement to forgo his or her right to privacy in sport are often ignored. When the only options available to elite athletes are to play by WADA's rules or to not play at all, the consent given by athletes may not be truly voluntarily or freely given. It is important to note that athletes waive their rights to privacy because doing otherwise implies guilt, a refusal to submit to testing and an automatic suspension from competing at the elite level of sport.

Beauchamp and Childress (2001, 297) point out that 'when individuals voluntarily grant others some form of access to themselves, their act is an *exercise* of the right to privacy, not a waiver of that right.... We exercise the right to privacy by reducing privacy in order to achieve other goals.' Despite whether athletes are exercising the right to privacy or waiving that right entirely when they consent to having samples of their urine, blood or tissues analysed for doping detection purposes, the fact that declining to provide a sample renders them guilty in the eyes of the sporting world, and particularly the Court of Arbitration for Sport, is problematic. If Moore (2000, 105) is correct that 'controlling who has access to ourselves is an essential part of being a happy and free person', then one could not consider the wilful and mandatory violation of an athlete's right to privacy an acceptable rule to legislate in sport.

Sport-governing bodies hold considerable power over those who want to compete in the events they organise and run. Some of the more troubling aspects of genetic enhancement and doping detection rules are espoused in the statement: 'I am not so worried about the prospects of a brave new world brought upon us by gene manipulation – I am much more worried when societies, committees, and concerned citizens use the force of government to tell us what we can do to and in our own bodies' (Moore 2000, 98). In the context of sport, this speaks to the rules that the athletes must adhere to if they wish to participate and the methods they are told they can and cannot use in their quests for athletic success. Athletes make many sacrifices on their way to joining the ranks of the best in the world in their chosen disciplines, and allowing their privacy to be violated by doping detection tests appears to be only one of the many questionable choices athletes are forced to make on their way to athletic superstardom.

Athletes might feel that the end results of Olympic medals and international success justify the means taken to achieve these feats. The consequentialist argument that the rewards of social justice outweigh the costs and consequences of potential privacy violations can be very persuasive (Farrelly 2002). Some athletes might think the creation of 'clean' and doping-free sport balances the privacy losses they sustain in providing samples and having their results reported to the public. It is possible that athletes who think this way have been taught to do so over the numerous years they have spent training and following the orders of coaches and sport-governing bodies. An athlete in this group might become accustomed to adhering to rules without first engaging in critical reflection or considering the implications of his or her actions outside the sporting world. Similarly, others have argued that despite the acceptance of random drug-testing as part of the culture of elite sport, the privacy rights violated by these tests are unacceptable from the deontological and existentialism positions and are only tentatively acceptable from the utilitarian point of view even if the tests are proven to be effective in combating doping in sport (Malloy and Zakus 2000).

Genetic testing and detection in sport is obviously plagued with moral concerns. The Privacy Commissioner of Canada's report, *Genetic Testing and Privacy*, includes the astute observation that there is a

> parallel between unlocking the gene in the '90s and unlocking the atom in the '40s. In both cases the excitement of discovery dulled critical assessment of the implications. In both cases we allowed scientists to unleash forces which can alter life as we know it, paid for their efforts with public funds and, at least initially, set few ethical or legal control on the enterprises. (Privacy Commissioner of Canada 1990, 3)

The Canadian Privacy Commissioner's companion document, *Drug Testing and Privacy*, bluntly acknowledges that drug testing constitutes an invasion of privacy noting, 'the principle privacy issue flowing from drug testing is not whether it is intrusive. It is' (Privacy Commissioner of Canada 1992, 22). As such, it is crucial to establish under what circumstances testing can be considered a justifiable action. These sentiments are echoed in the observation that 'regardless of which definition of privacy one tends to accept there is little doubt that drug testing is an invasion of privacy. The critical question is when can this invasion be justified?' (Malloy and Zakus 2000, 210)

Indeed, this is an important question in sport, and it is one that ethicists working with WADA must address. In attempting to justify the use of drug testing in sport, the Canadian government acknowledges, 'while there is no doubt that drug testing infringes personal privacy in a profound sense, one must not be blind to the need to protect the public interest' (Privacy Commissioner of Canada 1992, 3). In Canada, concerns of social justice apparently outweigh individuals' rights to privacy in contexts where drug testing is considered acceptable, such as in tests carried out by the national parole board and the department of national defence. It is not clear why sport is included among these ranks and a defensible position is lacking. Weighing the pros and cons of drug testing and privacy, or more broadly liberty and public interest, is not and never has been an easy task, but it is one that requires immediate attention if WADA plans to add genetic testing to its doping detection repertoire.

The extent that testing for genetic enhancements infringes athletes' rights to privacy should not be taken lightly. Both the method of conducting random unannounced testing and the requirement that athletes supply their whereabouts at all times, so that anti-doping agencies will be able to locate them in order to conduct doping tests, are indicative of the lack of concern given to athletes' privacy. Murray (2002) argues that athletes do not mind the invasion of privacy that comes with being tested for banned substances because it ensures that their opponents will not gain unfair advantages. Yet the counterargument that athletes cannot refuse to take a doping test without punishment renders the voluntariness of their consent suspect and cannot be ignored.

Nonetheless, athletes accept that the rules of sport are concrete and neither malleable nor optional. All competitors face the same standardised conditions when participating in elite sport and all must subject themselves to the full range of tests WADA deems necessary to ensure elite sport is as fair as possible. A more democratic method of making rules might make impositions on athletes' rights to privacy easier to justify and is an issue that requires further study. Clashes between technology and privacy 'seek a solution in which the technology does not dictate the extent of privacy protection' (DeCew 1999, 254). It remains to be seen how much knowledge athletes have of the notions of informed consent and coercion, or how much freedom they will have to opt in or out of genetic-testing measures.

But for now we are left with the following conundrum: detection requires testing to identify doping violations in sport; testing requires access to athletes' genetic information; and accessing genetic information creates many potential privacy issues and concerns throughout the world. Detecting genetic enhancements in sport using genetic tests is thus problematic and lacks a simple solution. Sport-governing bodies will face a serious problem if genetic tests are introduced to identify genetic modifications because the available and foreseeable detection methods demand athletes give up a considerable amount of privacy. If bans on genetic modifications remain in place, we are obligated to find a morally acceptable way of addressing this problem to ensure that, doped or not, athletes are treated as autonomous human beings worthy of privacy and respect.

ACKNOWLEDGEMENTS

I would like to thank Claudio Tamburrini and Angela Schneider for their helpful feedback on earlier drafts of this paper, and Christian Munthe and Mike McNamee for their challenging questions and comments at the 'Legitimate and illegitimate enhancements, where to draw the line?' conference, which I have since incorporated into this paper.

NOTES

1. See, for instance, Alfino and Mayes 2003, 1–18, and Beckman 2005, 97.
2. There are, of course, also significant differences between the roles female athletes are pressured to embody and adhere to and the expectations placed on male athletes. These gender differences manifest themselves in the different conception many people hold of the ideal female athlete compared to the ideal male athlete. However, this paper discusses

athletes as one group with respect to privacy issues without dividing the category of athlete into female athletes and male athletes.

3. Despite the lack of consensus on a definition of privacy, several scholars agree it is useful to separate issues pertaining to privacy of the person from issues of information privacy when examining a particular application of privacy. The former involves respecting the boundary between a person and the world to enable people to embrace their personhood, autonomy and identity, whereas the latter involves respecting an individual's privacy by not acquiring knowledge about that individual without their consent. Related terminology divides the concept into its spatial and informational dimensions, where spatial privacy refers to a person's private spaces that others are forbidden from accessing without permission, such as one's home and body, and informational privacy refers to preventing others from releasing details about one's life to the public. See, for instance, Parrot et al. 1989, 1381; Woogara 2005, 274; and Beckman 2005, 98.

4. See, for instance, Parker 2002, 103, and Taylor 2002, 588.

5. Pound made this remark in Seattle, Washington, at the annual meeting of the American Association for the Advancement of Science (AAAS) on 11 February 2004 and has repeated similar sentiments in several televised interviews in Canada since then. See http://www.wada-ama.org/en/newsarticle.ch2?articleId=188938 for the full transcript of his remarks.

6. For a thorough discussion of the elements of informed consent as they apply to genetic testing in sport, see Munthe 2005, 119–20.

REFERENCES

ADAM, D. 2001. Gene therapy may be up to speed for cheats at 2008 Olympics. *Nature* 414 (6): 569–70.

ALFINO, M. and G.R. MAYES. 2003. Reconstructing the right to privacy. *Social Theory and Practice* 29 (1): 1–18.

BEAUCHAMP, T. and J. CHILDRESS. 2001. *Principles of Biomedical Ethics.* 5th edn, New York: Oxford University Press.

BECKMAN, L. 2005. Democracy and genetic privacy: The value of bodily integrity. *Medicine, Health Care and Philosophy* 8: 97–103.

BROCKETT, P.L. and E.S. TANKERSLEY. 1997. The genetics revolution, economics, ethics and insurance. *Journal of Business Ethics* 16: 1661–76.

DECEW, J.W. 1999. Alternatives for protecting privacy while respecting patient care and public health needs. *Ethics and Information Technology* 1: 249–55.

———. 2004. Privacy and policy for genetic research. *Ethics and Information Technology* 6: 5–14.

FARRELLY, C. 2002. Genes and social justice: A Rawlsian reply to Moore. *Bioethics* 16 (1): 72–83.

FRASER, A.D. 2004. Doping control from a global and national perspective. *Therapeutic Drug Monitoring* 26 (2): 171–4.

HAYRAY, M. and T. TAKALE. 2001. Genetic information, rights, and autonomy. *Theoretical Medicine* 22: 403–14.

HONOUR, J.W. 2004. The fight for fair play. *Nature* 430: 143–4.

MCARTHUR, R.L. 2001. Reasonable expectations of privacy. *Ethics and Information Technology* 3 (2): 123–8.

MCCRORY, P. 2003. Super athletes or gene cheats? *British Journal of Sports Medicine* 37 (3): 192–3.

MALCOLM, H.A. 2005. Does privacy matter? Former patients discuss their perceptions of privacy in shared hospital rooms. *Nursing Ethics* 12 (2): 156 – 66.

MALLOY, D.C. and D.H. ZAKUS. 2000. Ethics of drug testing in sport – an invasion of privacy justified? *Sport, Education and Society* 7 (2): 203 – 18.

MIAH, A. 2004. *Genetically Modified Athletes.* London and New York: Routledge.

MOORE, A.D. 2000. Owning genetic information and gene enhancement techniques: Why privacy and property rights may undermine social control of the human genome. *Bioethics* 14 (2): 97 – 119.

———. 2003. Privacy: Its meaning and value. *American Philosophical Quarterly* 40 (3): 215 – 27.

MUNTHE, C. 2005. Ethics of controlling genetic doping. In *Genetic Technology and Sport: Ethical Questions,* edited by C. Tamburrini and T. Tännsjö. Abingdon and New York: Routledge: 107 – 25.

MURRAY, T.H. 2002. Reflections on the ethics of genetic enhancement. *Genetics in Medicine* 4 (6 Supplement): 27S – 32S.

PARKER, L.S. 2002. Information(al) matters: Bioethics and the boundaries of the public and the private. *Social Philosophy & Social Foundation* 19 (2): 83 – 112.

PARROT, R., J.K. BURGOON, M. BURGOON and B.A. LEPOIRE. 1989. Privacy between physicians and patients: More than a matter of confidentiality. *Social Science & Medicine* 29: 1381 – 5.

PASCUAL, J.A., V. BELALCAZAR, C. DE BOLOS, R. GUTIÉRREZ, E. LLOP and J. SEGURA. 2004. Recombinant Erythropoietin and analogues: A challenge for doping control. *Therapeutic Drug Monitoring* 26 (2): 175 – 9.

POUND, R. 2004. Remarks by WADA President Richard W. Pound at AAAS annual meeting. Available at http://www.wada-ama.org/en/newsarticle.ch2?articleId=188938, accessed 10 April 2007.

PRIVACY COMMISSIONER OF CANADA. 1990. *Genetic Testing and Privacy.* Ottawa: Minister of Supply and Services Canada.

———. 1992. *Drug Testing and Privacy.* Ottawa: Minister of Supply and Services Canada.

SCHNEIDER, A.J. 2005. Genetic enhancement of athletic performance. In *Genetic Technology and Sport: Ethical Questions,* edited by C. Tamburrini and T. Tännsjö. Abingdon and New York: Routledge: 32 – 41.

SCHNEIDER, A.J. AND R.B. BUTCHER. 2001. An ethical analysis of drug testing. In *Doping in Elite Sport: The Politics of Drugs in the Olympic Movement,* edited by W. Wilson and E. Derse. Champaign-Urbana, IL: Human Kinetics: 129 – 52.

SCHNEIDER, A.J. and T. FRIEDMANN 2006. *Gene Doping in Sports: The Science and Ethics of Genetically Modified Athletes.* Boston, MA: Elsevier Academic Press.

TAYLOR, J.S. 2002. Privacy and autonomy: A reappraisal. *Southern Journal of Philosophy* 40: 587 – 603.

THOMSON, J.J. 1975. The Right to Privacy. *Philosophy & Public Affairs* 4: 295 – 314.

THOMPSON, P.B. 1995. Privacy and the urinalysis testing of athletes. In *Philosophic Inquiry in Sport,* edited by W.J. Morgan and K.V. Meier. Champaign-Urbana, IL: Human Kinetics: 313 – 18.

VOLKMAN, R. 2003. Privacy as life, liberty, property. *Ethics and Information Technology* 5 (4): 199 – 210.

WARREN, S.D. and L.D. BRANDEIS. 1890. The right to privacy. *Harvard Law Review* 4: 193 – 220.

WOLFORTH, B., M.S. BRAY, J.M. HAGBERG, L. PÉRUSSE, R. RAURAMAA, M.A. RIVIERA, S.M. ROTH, T. RANKINEN and C. BOUCHARD. 2005. The human gene map for performance and health-related fitness phenotypes: The 2004 update. *Medicine and Science in Sports and Exercise* 37 (6): 881 – 903.

WOOGARA, J. 2005. Patients' privacy of the person and human rights. *Nursing Ethics* 12 (3): 273 – 87.

WORLD ANTI-DOPING AGENCY. 2003. *World Anti-Doping Code*. Montreal: World Anti-Doping Agency.

GENETIC ENHANCEMENT, SPORTS AND RELATIONAL AUTONOMY

Susan Sherwin

This paper explores the question of what attitude we should take towards efforts to develop the technology required to allow genetic enhancement of individuals in order to improve performance in sports: specifically, should we (a) welcome such innovations, (b) resign ourselves to their inevitable appearance or (c) actively resist their development and widespread adoption? Much of the literature on this topic leans towards options (a) or (b). I argue against both (a) and (b) and appeal to the concept of relational autonomy in support of option (c). I argue that we should situate the debate as a question of social policy rather than simply a matter for individual choice.

Resumen

Este artículo explora la pregunta sobre qué actitud debemos tomar con respecto a los esfuerzos para desarrollar la tecnología requerida para permitir la mejora genética de individuos con vistas a incrementar el rendimiento deportivo: específicamente, ¿deberíamos (a) dar la bienvenida a tales innovaciones, (b) resignarnos a su aparición inevitable, o (c) resistir activamente su desarrollo y amplia adopción? Una gran parte de la literatura sobre este tema se inclina por las opciones (a) o (b). Yo discuto contra ambas (a) y (b) y aludo al concepto de autonomía relacional para apoyar la opción (c). Argumento que debemos presentar el debate como una cuestión de política social en vez de simplemente como un asunto de elección personal.

Zusammenfassung

Dieser Artikel geht der Frage nach, welche Position zu beziehen sei gegenüber den gentechnischen Bestrebungen zur Verbesserung der individuellen Leistungsfähigkeit im Sport: genauer gefragt, sollten wir (a) derartige Besterbungen willkommen heißen, (b) uns mit der Unvermeidbarkeit ihres Daseins abfinden, oder (c) aktiv der Entwicklung und Weiterverbreitung entgegentreten? Ein Großteil der themenrelevanten Literatur tendiert zu den Optionen (a) oder (b). Ich argumentiere gegen (a) und (b) und unterstütze in Bezug auf das Konzept der Selbstbestimmung Option (c). In meiner Argumentation spreche ich mich für die Behandlung dieser Debatte im Rahmen der Gesellschaftspolitik aus und weniger als Frage der persönlicher Entscheidungen.

摘要

本文旨在探討，為了增進運動的表現，在努力發展能允許個人基因提升的科技中，我們應採取什麼樣的態度？特別而言，我們是應該採取（a）歡迎此項變革，（b）順從此項不可避免的現象，或者（c）積極反對此項新科技的發展與廣泛的被採納。大部分和此議題相關的文獻，不是傾向（a）就是（b），我反對此二者，並呼籲支持（c）的立場。所持的理由是，我們應該將此爭論置放在社會政策的層面，而非簡單地將此視為個人選擇的課題。

In 1973, the Canadian Public Health Association produced a 15-second television public service announcement that showed a 60-year-old Swede jogging effortlessly beside a puffing 30-year-old Canadian. The image was striking and it became permanently ingrained in the consciousness of Canadians of my generation. The intention was to shame us into becoming more active by demonstrating what was possible in a more fitness-conscious culture. Some of us, however, looked at our own ageing, short, overweight parents and predicted that no amount of exercise would compensate for our non-Swedish genetic heritage. In direct counterpoint to the explicit message that exercise leads to fitness, a more subtle subtext was also conveyed, namely that fitness requires 'good genes'.

Today, we seem to be moving closer to being able to 'correct' for an unathletic genetic heritage, perhaps even to being able to improve on an already very good genetic endowment through interventions of genetic enhancement. In this paper, I explore the question of what attitude we should take towards efforts to develop the necessary technology: specifically, should we (a) welcome such innovations, (b) resign ourselves to their inevitable appearance or (c) actively resist their development and widespread adoption? In addressing this question, I will argue, we must decide whether to situate the debate as a question of social policy or as a matter for individual choice.

Much of the literature on this topic leans towards options (a) or (b): indeed, some option (a) enthusiasts can hardly wait for the arrival of genetic enhancement technology and urge us to welcome it with open arms,[1] while other, more cautious (b) types argue that genetic enhancement technology is inevitable so we might as well accept it and concentrate on the details as to how it will be rolled out (see, for example, Baylis and Robert 2004). It is my intention to argue against both of these strategies and in favour of option (c), i.e. that we should actively resist the development and widespread adoption of this technology. First, though, I shall explain why I oppose the first two options.

My objections are based on pragmatic, health, and moral grounds. I have grave doubts about the safety, accuracy, and ultimate value of the entire research programme aimed at genetic enhancement, especially for the sake of improved athletic performance (rather than to avoid serious illness or disability). For one thing, the specific objectives of genetic enhancement for sports are vague, since it is by no means clear what we should wish to modify to improve performance in sports. While it seems likely that genes have an impact on body size and type and that these features are important considerations for many sports, we must be mindful that ideal body shapes vary by sport. Bodies that are desirable for weightlifting or sumo wrestling are likely to be problematic for anyone interested in track, gymnastics or soccer, while bodies that are well suited to high jumping may be a disadvantage to anyone aspiring to a career in ice hockey. By the same token, long limbs may be very helpful for basketball players but a virtual disqualification for women keen on ice dancing.

Moreover, although most sports involve a significant psychological element, it may not always be the same element. I imagine that athletes in all sports benefit from an ability to concentrate and a temperament that allows them to invest long hours in disciplined practice, but there may be a fine line between having the focused discipline needed for a successful training regime and being afflicted with a clinical obsessive-compulsive disorder. Such complexities would make it difficult to calibrate the necessary temperamental inclinations. And while some sports (e.g. golf) require a propensity for independent action, others (e.g. American football) demand a willingness to follow the strategic direction of others. In addition, even though most sports require a strong sense of competition, some (e.g. bicycle racing) demand an equally strong sense of cooperation and self-sacrifice.

When we think about genetic enhancement for sports, then, we must be careful about what, precisely, is desired. Given the wide diversity of sports and the complex demands of each, there is no clear single trait (or traits) that would constitute an advantage for every sport. Which genetic traits we would seek in order to 'enhance' an individual's ability to compete successfully would surely depend on what sport that particular person fancies. This suggests that the timing of genetic enhancement should be relatively late in an individual's life in order to allow the person to determine what particular sport (if any) is of personal interest; which means that it would be inappropriate to perform such interventions in the prenatal or infancy period when they would likely have the greatest impact. Presumably, enhancements would be carried out during adolescence, once preferences have begun to emerge and when there is still time to make a significant change in the individual; unfortunately, this is already a period of great bodily, psychological and emotional transformations and it is far from an ideal time for such weighty decisions. I will return to this point later.

Another reason to object to efforts to develop genetic interventions aimed at improving athletic performance is that, if we are not careful, we will reverse the intended message of the 1973 Canadian fitness campaign and promote the counter-message of the subtext: it seems all too easy to convince people that genes are, indeed, such a crucial element for fitness or athletic success that those with 'imperfect' genetic composition need not even bother to try to engage in athletic endeavours. The enthusiasm for genetic modification conveys popular, but false, reductionist assumptions of genetic determinism that suggest that genes are, quite literally, destiny. Although scientists who work on genetic modifications readily acknowledge that genes must be expressed and that their specific expression is determined by the environment(s) in which they occur, scientists have not done nearly enough to discourage popular discussion of various genes as if they translate directly into specific traits independently of their environment (e.g. the view that with the right genes, one can expect to be tall, smart, strong, courageous and well-coordinated no matter what the physical and social environment). Yet, even if I am able to acquire the genes necessary to build larger muscle mass, if I lack money to hire a trainer, if

I am terrified of being hurt, if I dislike undressing in the locker-room at the gym or if I lack balance, I will not be anyone's 'million dollar baby'. Clearly, genetic enhancement alone can be no guarantee of athletic success.

Hence I am deeply sceptical about the scientific prospects of developing and implementing a safe and reliable programmme of precise genetic enhancements for sports. I do not think the scientists engaged in related work are anywhere near being able to do such a thing, and I believe that whatever genetic modifications scientists might eventually learn how to achieve will be of questionable value. Of course, I may be wrong about this, and if I am – that is, if genetic enhancements really do prove effective in making a significant difference in athletic performance – then we can assume that the strongly competitive environment of most sports will drive elite (and not so elite) athletes to pursue the relevant modifications along with any other techniques that might improve their competitive advantage. As such, these types of intervention will probably soon become widespread and, therefore, of relatively little advantage to any single user. Either way, the risk-benefit ratio seems certain to be low for those who employ this technology.

Moreover, before the technology can be marketed, it will need to be subjected to large-scale clinical trials involving both adult and child subjects. It seems, though, that the outcome of the required research programme will serve no significant personal or social goods (beyond possibly providing an advantage to a few early users and generating some personal or corporate profit). In other words, it is unlikely that the research results would serve a sufficiently important good as to justify accepting the individual and social risks inherent in its development. It follows that the process of development would constitute a poor use of scarce research resources (money, trained researchers, human volunteers). For all these reasons, then, it will (or, at least, it should) be impossible to obtain approval from a responsible research ethics board to conduct the human trials that would be necessary before offering genetic enhancements for improving athletic performance to the public.

Given the serious problems associated with all aspects of the enterprise, we ought to avoid option (a) and refrain from enthusiastically welcoming these types of genetic interventions. In the absence of strong evidence that mastering genetic enhancement for sports would represent an important public good, the case against heading down this path in the first place is far stronger than the argument in its favour. We should, therefore, reject option (a).

For similar reasons, I believe we should also reject option (b), where, even though we lack enthusiasm for these sorts of genetic interventions, we resign ourselves to their inevitable appearance and simply try to control the conditions of their use. In other words, option (b) would have us treat genetic enhancements like steroid use and other forms of questionable drug use in athletics. Although my deep scepticism about the reliability of efforts at genetic enhancement calls into question the assumption that their development is inevitable, my cynicism suggests that the existence of significant scientific and moral obstacles to production of this technology may not be enough to make the issue go away. Inevitability theorists are probably correct on one matter: popular belief in the effectiveness of genetic enhancements will lead to a growing clamour for access regardless of the lack of evidence regarding their likely benefits or indication of foreseeable risks. As we have seen, many other products that purport to improve athletic performance have been snatched up by eager sports consumers without proof of either safety or effectiveness.

I am willing to allow that I may be wrong in my empirical predictions about the actual effectiveness of this project; I acknowledge that it may eventually prove possible to improve sports performance through genetic enhancement. In that case, genetic interventions will likely constitute the next form of 'doping' and producers will surely find willing consumers no matter how uncertain the scientific value or how high the risks. Many athletes find the rewards of winning irresistible and we must assume they will accept (even demand) all products that might improve their own personal prospects. Genetic modifications may prove impossible to test for and, therefore, impossible to regulate. As I shall explain below, once the genie is out of the bottle, the pressure on athletes may become unacceptable. I shall argue that if this were to occur, the resulting transformation of sport would likely be undesirable. Resigned acceptance is not an adequate response to the foreseeable, and undesirable, cultural shift associated with introduction of this technology. Therefore, option (b), should be rejected along with option (a). We should neither welcome nor accept development and introduction of genetic modifications for the sake of enhancing performance in sports.

This leaves us with option (c), or active resistance. Unlike inevitability theorists, I believe that we do, collectively, have the power to resist this research programme – though it will, undoubtedly, require a great deal of political effort to establish the necessary international agreements. In order to generate the necessary political engagement to support a policy of resistance, it will surely be necessary to do more than simply challenge the other two alternatives (enthusiasm and reluctant acceptance). The political support required for an effective strategy of resistance must be grounded in persuasive positive ethical arguments.

I shall, therefore, outline two interrelated arguments in support of the option of active resistance to development of this technology. Both arguments require that we reflect on the second question that I posed – i.e. we must decide whether to situate the debate as a question of social policy or as a matter for individual choice. I shall argue that the development and availability of genetic enhancements must be framed as a matter of social policy, not individual choice. The first step in making the case against permitting development of genetic enhancement in sports is to dispose of the counter-argument that urges us to respect individual choice, equated with autonomy, in this area. According to the free choice argument, we should allow individual users to decide if they wish to accept the risks involved in genetic modification, provided that they have available full and accurate information about the risks and benefits involved. The respect for the individual choice position is rooted in traditional understandings about the autonomy rights of individuals. My response to this argument will be that we need to supplant traditional interpretations of autonomy with a relational alternative. A relational approach to autonomy will make clear that respect for autonomy does not require us to enable consumer access to this technology.

Before sketching a relational version of autonomy, I shall review the familiar argument in favour respecting individual choice. Given the promises attached to genetic modification technology, and the very high rewards often attached to winning athletic competitions, we can anticipate that some (aspiring) athletes – or perhaps some parents – will want access to the specific interventions involved. These would-be consumers will make a strong demand for freedom of choice regarding its use. Maximum personal freedom is a cornerstone of the liberal political theories that inform the workings of modern democratic states; it is widely believed that individuals are best served by being granted the most extensive liberty possible. According to this view, so long as the technology proves to be not excessively dangerous, we should interpret autonomy as demanding that individuals be allowed to make their own informed decisions about using it.

There are, however, important pragmatic grounds for challenging rights-based claims to the use of genetic enhancement technologies for sports. The most important of these is that recognition of such a right for some is likely to result in reduced autonomy for others. This is because the practice of sports is inherently a competitive activity. Whenever it is learned (or suspected) that some of the leaders in a sport are benefiting from a particular product or training technique, many others will follow suit in an effort to improve or at least maintain their own standing. Whatever form of technology seems to offer an improved competitive edge, no matter how slight, is quickly taken up by competitors, be it clothing design, instruments of performance (e.g. golf clubs, football shoes, bicycles) or training techniques. It is easy to witness this pattern in other biological programmes such as the use of steroids in baseball, blood doping in biking or marijuana in snowboarding. Thus, at the elite level, it may be that some athletes can and will make an informed, autonomous decision to use genetic enhancement, but if those athletes are successful, their competitors will find their own range of meaningful options reduced: they will feel compelled to employ genetic modification themselves or give up on elite competition. Surely, though, autonomy must include a meaningful right to refuse as well as to adopt a technology. In this case, the freedom to resist use of the technology will likely be very hollow – better described as a narrowing of most athletes' overall autonomy than as a protection of it. This is not (yet) an argument against allowing individuals to choose genetic enhancement technologies; rather, the argument is meant to make clear that we should not feel bound by the simple appeal that we must respect an individual's right to autonomously choose to use such a technology.

To make the stronger argument against allowing individuals the opportunity to choose this technology we need to reflect more deeply upon the very nature of autonomy. We can begin this task by recognising that the problem of reduced autonomy for all but the initial users will not be restricted to a small cadre of elite world-class athletes. There is likely to be a significant trickle-down effect on aspiring young athletes who hope to qualify for athletic scholarships or professional sports careers. In fact, as noted above, genetic interventions will probably be deployed no later than adolescence, when both body and mind are still taking shape and are malleable to desired modifications. While the freedom to refuse is likely to be limited for all competitors, when the interventions must occur during adolescence (or earlier) – i.e. at a time when risk-taking is especially high and mature reasoning rare, when hormones, body shape and brain are undergoing rapid and disorienting changes, when peer pressure weighs especially heavily and when undesirable side effects might be especially damaging – it is very misleading to describe individual choices regarding the use of this technology as an expression of personal liberty. In fact, respecting autonomy as the ability to live in accordance with one's deepest values and interests would seem to require us to limit the opportunities for adolescents to undertake genetic modifications that pose risks to their long-term health and potential, just as we now try to limit their risk-taking behaviour in the realms of tobacco, alcohol, steroids and drug use. By protecting vulnerable adolescents from risky short-term behaviours, society strives to increase their options for greater autonomy and a better range of life choices in the future. Similar reasoning would apply to the use of genetic enhancement technologies if they ever do reach the market.

We can see, then, that autonomy is not simply a question of not interfering with an individual's preferences. If we are to respect autonomy as a moral principle with relevance to the question of access to genetic enhancement technologies aimed at athletic performance, we must understand its complex social nature so that we can support policies that promote overall autonomy throughout a lifetime. I shall say more about the social nature of autonomy below. For now, let us agree that when autonomy is understood as consumer freedom, the argument in favour of free access fails on its own terms, since unconstrained consumer freedom ultimately leads to less overall autonomy for most prospective athletes.

There is a further, and deeper, reason to challenge the individualistic ethical framework that threatens to lead us down this slippery slope into widespread use of genetic enhancement technologies in sport (and elsewhere). To explain the second reason to object to this framework, I will need to sketch out a conceptual argument for rejecting traditional autonomy defences in general and for adopting a social policy framework instead. In particular, I propose that we reject individualistic interpretations of autonomy and personhood and supplant them with relational understandings of these core concepts. Elsewhere, I have made more extensive arguments for this shift, so here I will offer only a brief summary of the implications of relational theory to the current debate.[2]

Relational theory, as I pursue it, rejects the dominant ideal of persons as independent, rational, self-interested deliberators who are ontologically prior to society. Instead, it conceives of persons as (at least partially) constituted by social interactions. Relational persons are more complex and less transparent than are the persons of most liberal individualist theories. Where liberal theories treat selfhood as a unified state with well-ordered, rational preferences accessible to the agent, relational accounts understand selfhood to be an ongoing project in which different aspects of the self may be in tension with one another – a situation that complicates the meaning of autonomy. Relational theorists deny that people typically discover their own values by introspection and support the view that persons *determine* their values through dialogue with others and action. Since values are *formed through* social engagement (rather than prior to it), we should not focus on the question 'what does a person want to do now?' but rather on 'what are the processes by which he/she has come to hold his current preferences?' and 'are the meaningful options before him/her ones that are supportive of his overall interests?' Addressing these latter questions requires us to step back and examine the social conditions under which particular options are developed and made salient while others are eclipsed as irrelevant in the current climate. On a relational account, autonomy involves more than a single agent making a particular isolated decision. It involves consideration of the types of choices facing agents and the forces that may be structuring those choices. Hence, autonomy requires more than an ability to make a rational informed choice – it also requires a social context that does not encourage selection of options that are contrary to an agent's overall well-being (and are within the realm of society's ability to support).

Feminist theory has helped to reveal how social conditions can distort an individual's ability to pursue options that support her interests. Specifically, feminists have shown how oppression produces social conditions that make compliance with oppressive norms the most reasonable option available to individuals (see, for example, MacKenzie and Stoljar 2000). For example, a society that rewards beautiful women and punishes those considered ugly creates conditions that make it 'irrational' for women in the latter category to choose not to seek cosmetic surgery despite the costs, risks or anxiety such surgery involves. It is the rational choice of an informed consumer even though widespread use of cosmetic surgery to promote conformation with oppressive beauty norms undermines women's ultimate equality by reinforcing the view that a socially approved appearance is of fundamental importance for women. Moreover, as more and more women rely on surgery to alter their appearance, the demands of 'normalcy' become ever more elusive to 'average' women; as a result, women feel social pressure to undergo (often repeated) surgical modification.

Moreover, oppression is not the only condition that generates such problematic outcomes. There are many types of circumstances where the immediate interest of individuals is contrary to their collective long-term well-being. A similar pattern is evident in the giant tragedy of the commons of our planet, in that what appears to be rational and reasonable for an individual to do regarding personal fossil-fuel and fresh-water consumption generates a terrible threat to the welfare of all. To reverse, or even to slow down, global warming we need collective action established through coordinated social policies – otherwise our distinct, personal, short-term interests will continue to threaten our overall well-being. Leaving decision-making about personal consumption of finite and polluting resources to individual agents acting rationally in their personal circumstances leads us down a path few of us would choose. These examples make vivid the need to understand autonomy as involving social conditions that make available meaningful options that support the overall interests of individuals rather than thinking only in terms of the immediate advantage of an isolated choice situation.

The use of genetic enhancement in sports (and elsewhere) seems certain to create a similar conundrum to the environmental complexity. As noted above, if this technology is actively pursued as a research programme to the point where use of such interventions becomes a realistic option for individuals seeking to improve their own performance, it may soon become irrational for serious competitors to refuse its use. At that point, we will find that we have done more than reduce the range of options for world-class athletes. We will also have changed the nature of sport, and even of humanity, in ways that may be detrimental to all. Winning will be the only continuing goal of sport and its pursuit could well eclipse other values attached to athletic activities, such as enjoyment, fitness, health, improved sense of self-esteem and excitement. Even spectators may find their interest and enjoyment sacrificed as they watch players who are increasingly alien to themselves. We will, thereby, deepen the notion that (athletic) success is best approached through strategic consumption of appropriate products; as well, we will very likely promote individualism and competitive values over solidarity and collective welfare. Such social transformations are contrary to the common good and the welfare of the majority of persons.

Moreover, such a programme of genetic modification for the sake of athletic success raises very profound questions about the nature of being human. Defining human excellence in terms that can be pursued through deliberate genetic modifications sends a clear message about the social value we attach to those who purchase the best technology (the 'winners') and also about the value we attach to those who are considered 'imperfect' or 'losers'. Once the genie of genetic enhancement for the sake of individual success is out of the bottle, it may not be long before we find ourselves in a world where such interventions are regarded as being just as normal and desirable as education and nutrition – just another means of personal 'improvement' and within the growing responsibilities of caring parents. In such an environment, it is difficult to imagine any of us feeling content with our own genetic makeup (or that of our partners, children or friends). What will be the expectations regarding personal self-help or 'self-improvement' and what will be a legitimate excuse for imperfection?

Use of this technology to generate a competitive advantage entrenches the legitimacy of competition among humans as a driving value for social policy. Social Darwinism makes it increasingly difficult, however, to pursue badly needed social programmes aimed at overall welfare and the urgent needs of the disadvantaged. Unrestricted genetic modifications represent more of the same, but they also signal the potential of particularly dramatic social changes. Moreover, there is simply no strong argument in favour of developing this technology which seems unlikely to serve any important personal or social goal. Apart from the potential profits foregone by producers and providers of genetic modification services, there are no significant opportunity costs to be lost in not developing the technology for use in sports. In the face of such serious social and personal risks – and in the absence of any clear social benefits or significant personal need – we should adopt the precautionary principle and hold off on developing this technology.

If it is human improvement or even human excellence we are after, we should not allow ourselves to be pushed down this slippery slope. Rather, we should pursue social programmes that will help to improve humanity through well-established social means. For example, public health programmes that will reduce the incidence and costs of disease, provide improved nutrition to poor children and avoid the widespread occurrence of disabling injuries from unregulated vehicles will result in more human beings achieving their full potential than any genetic enhancement programme likely would. In a similar vein, ensuring good educational and training opportunities to a larger segment of the world's population will result in many more people achieving excellence in their chosen pursuits. While less 'sexy' and less profitable than genetic modification strategies, social measures aimed at human improvement seem more likely to generate a world most humans can comfortably inhabit than those that encourage us to solve our personal limitations through technological alterations. Furthermore, even though it conflicts with simplistic interpretations of autonomy as informed consumer choice, it is the one policy that is supportive of the broadest range of individual autonomy understood relationally. Hence, I believe that the ethically appropriate response to the possibility of genetic modification for sport is (c), to adopt the option of active resistance to development and deployment of this technology.

ACKNOWLEDGEMENTS
I wish to thank Françoise Baylis, Richmond Campbell, Claudio Tamburrini and participants in the Dalhousie University philosophy department colloquium for their helpful comments on earlier drafts of this chapter.

NOTES

1. Transhumanists are amongst the most vocal enthusiasts. See their website at www.transhumanism.org.
2. This argument is spelled out much more fully in Sherwin 1998 and Sherwin 2003.

REFERENCES

BAYLIS, F. and J.S. ROBERT. 2004. The inevitability of genetic enhancement technologies. *Bioethics* 18 (1): 1–26.

MACKENZIE C. and N. STOLJAR, eds. 2000. *Relational Autonomy: Feminist Perspectives on Autonomy, Agency and the Social Self*. Oxford: Oxford University Press.

SHERWIN, S. 1998. A relational approach to autonomy in health care. In *The Politics of Women's Health: Exploring Agency and Autonomy*, edited by S. Sherwin, Francoise Baylis, Marilyn Bell, Maria De Koninck, Jocelyn Downie, Abby Lippman, Margaret Lock, Wendy Mitchinson, Kathryn Pauly Morgan, Janet Mosher, and Barbara Parish Philadelphia, PA: Temple University Press: 19–47.

———. 2003. The importance of ontology for feminist policy-making in the realm of reproductive technology. *Canadian Journal of Philosophy*, supp. vol. 26 (Feminist Moral Philosophy): 273–95.

WHOSE PROMETHEUS?
TRANSHUMANISM, BIOTECHNOLOGY
AND THE MORAL TOPOGRAPHY
OF SPORTS MEDICINE

Mike McNamee

The therapy/enhancement distinction is a controversial one in the philosophy of medicine, yet the idea of enhancement is rarely if ever questioned as a proper goal of sports medicine. This opens up latitude to those who may seek to use elite sport as a vehicle of legitimation for their nature-transcending ideology. Given recent claims by transhumanists to develop our human nature and powers with the aid of biotechnology, I sketch out two interpretations of the myth of Prometheus, in Hesiod and Aeschylus, which can help frame the moral limits of sports medicine. By way of conclusion I assemble some banal reminders: We are mortal beings; our vulnerability to disease, injury and the waning of our powers, far from something we can overcome or eliminate, represent natural limits both for morality and medicine generally and sports medicine in particular.

Resumen

La distinción entre terapía/amejoramiento físico es controvertida en la filosofía de la medicina, sin embargo la idea de la mejora ráramente, si acaso alguna vez, es cuestionada como un objetivo apropriado de la medicina deportiva. Esto deja márgen de acción a aquellos que busquen utilizar el deporte de élite como un vehículo que legitime su idelología de trascendencia de la naturaleza. Dadas ciertas reivindicaciones recientes por trashumanistas para desarrollar nuestra naturaleza humana y capacidades con la ayuda de la tecnología, boceto dos interpretaciones sobre el mito de Prometeo, en Hesíodo y Esquilo, que pueden ayudar a enmarcar los límites morales de la medicina deportiva. A modo de conclusión reuno algunos recordatorios banales: somos seres mortales; nuestra vulnerabilidad a la enfermedad, las lesiones, y el ocaso de nuestras capacidades, lejos de ser algo que podamos superar o eliminar, representan límites naturales para ambas, la moral y la medicina en general, y la medicina deportiva en particular.

Zusammenfassung

Die Unterscheidung zwischen Therapie und Leistungssteigerung wird in der Philosophie der Medizin kontrovers diskutiert, jedoch das Konzept der Leistungssteigerung als Ziel der

Sportmedizin wird selten hinterfragt. Dies eröffnet Handlungsspielräume für all jene, die den Leistungssport benutzen wollen, um ihre naturüberschreitende Ideologie zu legitimieren. Vor dem Hintergrund der aktuellen Aussagen von Transhumanisten, unsere menschliche Natur und Fähigkeiten mit Hilfe der Technik weiterentwickeln zu wollen, werde ich zwei Interpretationsmöglichkeiten der Prometheussage skizzieren (zum einen Hesiod und zum anderen Aischylos), um somit einen Betrachtungsrahmen für die moralischen Grenzen der Sportmedizin zu liefern. Die Auflistung elementarer Schlussfolgerungen soll diese Grenzen noch einmal in Erinnerung rufen: Wir sind sterbliche Wesen; unsere Anfälligkeit für Krankheiten, Verletzungen, sowie die Abnahme unsere Kräfte ist mit Nichten etwas was wir überwinden oder eliminieren können, sondern sie stellen natürliche Grenzen, sowohl für die moralische Betrachtung aus Sicht der Medizin im Allgemeinen, als auch der Sportmedizin im Besonderen dar.

摘要

在醫學哲學的研究中，治療/與增進表現之間的區別具有一種矛盾的現象。然而，增進表現的這個概念中很少被認為是運動醫學中所追求的適當目標。 這個觀點打開了一個自由空間來給那些想要使用頂尖運動來尋求做為一種合理 自然-超越 的意識型態。 基於最近的超人本主義者 (transhumanists) 觀點，經由科技的協助來發展我們的人性與權力，我勾勒出兩個有關 Promethus 神話 (Hesiod 與 Aeschylus) 的詮釋。 這兩個神話可幫助勾勒出運動醫學的限制。透過結論，我將一些老生長談的提示匯集起來： 我們是會死的人類；我們受制於疾病、傷害和衰老，這些是我們人類無法克服與免除的，這種易脆弱性代表著自然的限制，這在道德與醫學中，特別是在運動醫學上，是無法被克服或免除的。

1. Introduction

The rise of sports medicine to the apex of sports science is something that I believe has not been commented upon. There are hierarchies within hierarchies. Sports medicine sits over sports science which sits in panoramic ascendancy over what I take to be the humanities of sport: history, literature, philosophy and theology. I wish, against that hegemony, to challenge some of the more self-aggrandising possibilities of sports medicine. Its most recent incarnation is the image of 'genetically modified athletes'.[1] Recognising limits is not, however, a prominent feature of modern medicine. Indeed it is sometimes extremely unclear where medicine ends and other social practices such as social care, welfare or education begin.[2] If, however, this conceptual inflation spreads horizontally it effects a process widely referred to as the medicalisation of everyday life. It is not the sheer spread of medicine that concerns me here, but rather its vertical ambition in transforming our very nature as humans.

In a recent book, the American conservative bioethicist Leon Kass has written, somewhat polemically, that 'human nature itself lies on the operating table, ready for alteration, for eugenic and neuropsychic "enhancement", for wholesale design.

In leading laboratories, academic and industrial, new creators are confidently amassing their powers, while on the street their evangelists are zealously prophesying a posthuman future' (Kass 2004, 4). It is against this evangelising and self-promoting backdrop that I wish to problematise the unfettered application of science and technology to the sphere of sports medicine. To do this I wish first to note elements of science derived from the English philosopher, politician and polymath Sir Franics Bacon from the sixteenth and seventeenth centuries, which survive and in some sense shape the hubris of modern biomedical science. Secondly, I wish to challenge the assumptions of transhumanism, an ideology which seeks to complete the merely 'half-baked' project of human nature (Boström 2004). In response, I sketch out two interpretations of the myth of Promethus in Hesiod and Aeschylus which can help us see aright the moral limits of sports medicine. I conclude with a banal reminder: we are mortal beings. Our vulnerability to disease and death, far from something we can overcome or eliminate, represents natural limits both for morality and medicine generally and sports medicine in particular.

2. Baconian Science, Biomedical Technology and the Perfection of the Body

Though the ancient Greeks and, more generally, artists throughout history have had a deep and significant aesthetic respect for the perfection of human form, the obsession with physical perfectionism arises as a moral imperative, as sociologists of the body[3] have noted, with the increasing pervasiveness of modern technology. In the writings of Bacon, and also of Descartes, the impulse of experimental philosophy (conjoining the rational and the empirical) finds new expression in medical science. The allusion to the Baconian ideal itself belongs to Hans Jonas, whose railing against the hubris of medical technology prefigured much work in the fields of medical ethics and medical theology. Jonas wrote, as early as 1974, regarding the potential pitfalls of 'biological engineering'. Slightly, less rhetorically than Kass, he wrote that

> The biological control of man, especially genetic control, raises ethically questions of a wholly new kind for which neither previous praxis nor previous thought has prepared us. Since no less than the nature and image of man are at issue, prudence itself becomes our first ethical duty, and hypothetical reasoning our first responsibility. (Jonas 1974, 141)

It will be clear that the presence of Greek myths which raise in our imagination the proper limits of the human cast a shadow of doubt on the uniqueness of the controlling aspects of modern biology or genetics. And despite offering two contrasting lenses with which to view biotechnology, my own preference is marked by a precautionary stance. Moreover, I will claim in the final section that there is no need for the generation of a new ethics; rather that the moral sources for such evaluations as the proper ends of medicine and sports medicine themselves go back at least as far as Plato.

What is of particular interest, though, in the foundational drive for medical technologies in particular is one that fits with a very traditional conception of medicine as a healing art or as in the relief of suffering. The telos of such technology and its initial, moral, motivation is captured by Borgmann:

> The main goal of these programs seems to be the domination of nature. But we must be more precise. The desire to dominate does not just spring from a lust of power, from sheer human imperialism. It is from the start connected with the aim of liberating humanity from disease, hunger and toil, and of enriching life with learning, art and athletics. (Borgmann 1984, 36)

The relief of suffering is, of course one noble end associated with medicine traditionally conceived (Porter 2002; Cassell 2004; Edwards and McNamee 2006). But that is not the object of my concern, nor typically those of sports medics associated with elite sports. The idea is captured brilliantly in Gerald McKenny's excellent book on bioethics, technology and the body, *To Relieve the Human Condition* (1997). It is as if the fulfilment of science's quest for domination of nature was itself to culminate in overcoming *human* nature. Now, of course, the denial or denigration of human nature is not new: early behaviouristic psychology often included a claim that human nature was no more than a myth or a hangover from a pre-scientific age, and this ideology was given further impetus in the sociobiological movements of the 1980s. Nevertheless, modern science takes the body as an object in nature, capable of precise observation and minute description. The uses of science extend not merely to intervening in, but also to re-envisioning, the body. The rise of medical technology, however, opens entire new vistas for medicine as a social practice.

3. Technology in Medicine and Sports

It is easy to think of technology as a modern social practice and to assume a particular kind of technology (such as computer technology) to represent a paradigmatic example. Nye (2006) ties technology to tool-making but reminds us of the narratives in which our appreciation of those tools are rested. For example,

> In Herman Melville's *Moby Dick*, Queequeg, a South Sea harpooner visiting Nantucket, was offered a wheelbarrow to move his belongings from an inn to the dock. But he did not understand how it worked, and so, after putting all his gear into the wheel barrow he lifted it on to his shoulders. Most travellers have done something that looked equally silly to the natives, for we are all unfamiliar with some local technologies. This is another way of saying that we do not know the many routines and small narratives that underlie everyday life in other societies. (Nye 2006, 6)

This commonplace example is a reminder of the importance of locating our views of technology historically but also brings to mind a less manipulative conception than the kind which those opposed to radical biotechnologies conjure up as counter-examples. The term 'technology' has a venerable past. It derives from the conjoining of two Greek words *techne* and *logos*: *techne* refers to the kind of skill (practical knowledge) involved in making things, while by *logos* is meant a form of reasoning aimed at understanding the nature or form of things. Although we think of the term as a modern one, it was in fact first coined by Aristotle (Mitcham 1979) – but his meaning for it was the technical skills of rhetoric; literally the *techne* of *logos* (Kass 2002).

It is not uncommon, however, in everyday talk to slide the concept of science together with the concept of technology. Indeed, in the UK at least, sports scientists very often conflate their activities with what should properly be called sports technology.[4] Today philosophers of science clearly distinguish theory generation (science) and its application (technology), though the distinction is rather lost in the natural scientific study of sport. We could imagine then, that the domains of medical and sports technology might simply be taken to include the theoretical knowledge, practical knowledge and the instruments and products that bring about the ends of medicine or sports respectively. If this were acceptable, then their salient characteristic would be a 'means-end' structure. Technology might be thought of as the means utilised to pursue chosen ends. It would appear to follow, then, that technology is, in a sense, neutral. It is neither good nor bad *in itself*. Rather, its normativity is typically governed by the uses to which it is put. An example of this conceptualisation is found in the recent literature on philosophy of technology: 'Technology in its most robust sense ... involves the *invention, development, and cognitive deployment of tools and other artifacts, brought to bear on raw materials ... with a view to the resolution of perceived problems* ... which, together, allow [society] to continue to function and flourish' (Hickman 2001, 12). An equally sympathetic account is to be found in the UN Convention on Biological Diversity where biotechnology is defined thus: 'Biotechnology means any technological application that uses biological systems, living organisms, or derivatives thereof, to make or modify products or processes for specific use' (Article 2, Use of Terms).

Less authoratatively, and even more broadly, biotechnology can also be commonsensically defined thus: 'Biotechnology is the manipulation of organisms to do practical things and to provide useful products'.[5] While such global definitions are useful as a starting point, it is important to note that they fail to distinguish ethically important characteristics of different forms of practice that fall under the headings 'technology' or 'biotechnology'.

By contrast, then, a stronger line of criticism is found especially in continental European writers who have made problematic the assumption that technology is itself a neutral means to chosen (good or bad) ends. Mitcham (1995) gives an account of this history of technological scepticism in medicine (Kapp 1877; Dessauer 1927; Ortega y Gasset 1939; Heidegger 1977) and also notes more fundamental criticisms of technology as ideology where technology, far from being the handmaiden of man, comes full circle to be its master (Marcuse 1964; Habermas 1968; Foucault 1988). Although not as radical in her writings as these latter philosophers, Lee (2003) helpfully marks the following distinction in the application of science in the form of technology whose goals are: (1) explanation; (2) prediction; and (3) control.

It is the last of these aims that I want to pick up on in relation to any ethical evaluation of technologies. Nye, a historian of technology, arrives (far too swiftly for my liking) at a softer conclusion about the relations between technology and human kind. He writes: 'Stonehenge suggests the truth of Walter Benjamin's example that "technology is not the mastery of nature but of the relations between nature and man"' (Nye 2006, 7). Nevertheless, we find more classical sources that are to be interpreted less generously. Francis Bacon (1561 – 1626) is well known for his remarks on the development of scientific and technological methods whose aim would be 'to relieve man's estate' (i.e. of suffering/vulnerability), and likewise René Descartes (1596 – 1650) had wanted 'to use this knowledge ... for all the purposes for which it is appropriate, and thus make ourselves, as it were, the lords and masters of nature'. Of course, as C.S. Lewis pointed out in his essay, 'The abolition of man', every time we hear the phrase 'mastery of nature' we ought to be alerted to the fact that it is some particular group that is doing the mastering for its own reasons and in the light of its own version of the good, rather than the good of humanity (whatever that might look like).

Again, Lee distinguishes the types of control: (1) *weak*: avoid the occurrence; and (2) *strong*: prevent occurrence. And the facets comprising weak or strong control technological control of nature (or for my present concerns 'human nature') range from theoretical knowledge, through practical knowledge and skills, to instruments and products. Notwithstanding these cautionary considerations, I will consider biotechnology and sports technology respectively to refer to those technologies deployed to meet the ends or goals of sports medicine or sports respectively. What forms, more specifically, might this technology take? The most obvious uses by sports scientists and sports medics might be instrumentation such as hypoxic chambers (to assist the fastest recovery times for soft tissue and bone injuries[6]); gas analysers (to measure anaerobic contributions to exercise); and isokinetic strength testers or 'bod-pods' (to assess body density). Finally, the scourge of sports, many would say, fall into the category of 'technological products'. Most obvious here might be anabolic steroids or other doping supplements such as EPO or human growth hormone. Nevertheless, it is important to note that these products are often designed with medical therapies in mind. It is their use in the elite sports population that is problematic, not the nature of the products themselves.

What I want to do now is to step back a little from a discussion of the enhancement mantra that governs elite sports and some sections of what is called sports medicine and consider a broader and, to my mind, more problematic application of biotechnology to enhance human nature. It is an ideology that falls under the label 'transhumanism' (TH).[7] Rather than a unified entity, TH is a broad and heterogeneous group of thinkers who give technology a grander, Promethean, aim.

4. What (Good) is Transhumanism?

A range of views fall under the label of TH.[8] The most extreme is a view according to which TH is a project to overcome the inherent limitations of human nature. Examples of these limits, which most of us take for granted as part of the human condition, are appearance, life span and vulnerability to ageing, disease and so on. There is, however, a more extreme version of TH that sees the role of technology as one to vastly enhance both the person and his/her environment by exploiting a range of technologies including genetic engineering, cybernetics, computation and nanotechnology.

Recruitment of these various types of technology, it is hoped, will produce selves who are intelligent, immortal etc. but who are not members of the species *homo sapiens*. Their species type will be either be ambiguous, e.g. if they are cyborgs (part human, part machine). If they turn out to be wholly machines, they will lack any common genetic features with human beings. Extreme TH strongly supports such developments. Less extreme TH is satisfied to augment human nature with technology where possible and where desired by the individual.

At present TH seems to command support mostly in North America, though there are some adherents from Europe (see the website of the World Transhumanism Association). On one level it can be seen as an extension of neo-liberal or libertarian thought transferred into biomedical contexts. This is because the main driver appears to be the valorisation of autonomy as expressed in the economic choices of individuals. If certain technological developments enable greater defences against senescence, or if they can significantly enhance my powers of thought, speed and movement, then TH argues that anyone (as competent consumers) should be allowed to obtain them – if they can afford them, of course. Sandberg attempts to give an ethical underpinning to this essentially political programme. He argues that we must consider 'morphological freedom as a right' (Sandberg 2001).

Before TH is considered to be the product of outlandish free-thinkers who have enjoyed too much certain medico-technological products themselves, we must consider that it embodies two aims that are widely thought to be valued in the West. These are: (1) The use of technology to improve the lot of humans. Work in public health, e.g. construction of sewage systems, fluoride additives to water supplies to prevent dental decay and so on, is all work to facilitate this noble end that is shared with the entire medical enterprise. (b) The other widely shared value is that of increased autonomy such that the individual has greater scope in governing his own life-plan.

Moreover, proponents of TH say it presents an opportunity to plan the future development of human beings, the species *homo sapiens*. Instead of this being left to the evolutionary process and its exploitation of random mutations, TH presents a hitherto unavailable option, tailoring the development of human beings to an ideal blueprint. Typically educational, social and political reformers have been unable to carry forward their project with the kind of control and efficiency (it is said) that biologically driven technologies can.

5. Against Transhumanism

One can ascribe to Ellul a certain prescience: without knowledge of ideologies such as TH, he pointed out in 1965 that the development of technology will lead to a 'new dismembering and a complete reconstitution of the human being so that he can at least become the objective (and also the total object) of techniques' (Ellul 1965, 431). One possible consequence that can be read into the grander claims of some TH proponents is that, in effect, TH will lead to the existence of two distinct types of being, the human and the posthuman. The former are most likely to be viewed as some kind of underclass.

It is worth pursuing this argument a little. It is said that 'we' have a 'self-understanding' as human beings. This includes, for example, our essential vulnerability to disease, ageing and death. Parens (1995), in reversing the title of Nussbaum's celebrated book *The Fragility of Goodness*, captured this idea memorably when speaking of the 'goodness of fragility'. Suppose, however, that the strong TH project is realised. We are no longer so vulnerable, immortality is a real prospect. This will result in a change in our 'self-understanding'. This will have a normative element to it; most radically it may take the form of a change in what we view as a good life. Hitherto such a life this would have been assumed to be finite, but now this might change.

Habermas's (2003) objection can be interpreted more or less strongly. The strongest one is that *any* change in self-understanding is a morally bad thing. But this move is not a defensible one. Consider the changes in self-understanding that have occurred over the centuries: the advent of Christianity or Islam; the intellectual revolutions that preceded Copernicus; and Darwin. It does not follow necessarily that any particular change in self-understanding logically entails moral decline. There are many who would advocate that this constitutes not decline but rather moral progress.

There are, to my mind, more telling and less abstract arguments that can be marshalled effectively against TH. These concern, in the first place, a simple argument against inequality. The second relates to the unarticulated ends of TH. What is its telos? What do we enhance and why? Let us consider, albeit briefly, the first consideration.

Rather than considering two species of humanity, we might (perhaps crudely) consider the two categories of economics: the rich and the poor. The former can afford to make use of TH while the latter will not be able to. Given the commercialisation of elite sports, one can see both the attractions (for some) and the dangers here. Mere mortals – the unenhanced poor – will get no more than a glimpse of the transhuman in competitive elite sports contexts. There is, then, something of a double-binding character to this consumerism. The poor, at once removed from the possibility of choosing augmentation, end up paying for it by pay-per-view. The weak thus pay the strong for the pleasure of their envy. By contrast, one might see less corrosive aspects of this economically driven argument. Far from being worried about it, it might be said, TH is an irrelevance, since so few will be able to make use of the technological developments even if they ever manifest themselves.

Still further, critics point out that TH rests upon some conception of the good. As seen, for one group of TH advocates, the good is expansion of personal choice. But some critics object to what they see as consumerism of this kind. They suggest that the good cannot be equated with that which people choose. With regard to the other kind of TH proponents, those who see TH as an opportunity to enhance the general quality of life for humans, critics point out that this again presupposes some conception of the good, of what kind of traits are best to engineer into humans (disease-resistance, high intelligence etc.), and they disagree about precisely what 'objective goods' to try to select for installation into humans/posthumans. A further and stronger, though more abstract, objection is voiced by Habermas. This is that interfering with the process of human conception, and by implication human constitution, deprives humans of the 'naturalness which so far has been a part of the taken-for-granted background of our self-understanding as a species' and that 'Getting used to having human life at the biotechnologically enabled disposal of our contingent preferences cannot help but change our normative self-understanding' (Habermas 2003, 72). And will those TH agents (athletes and non-athletes alike), genetically and technologically modified to their autonomous heart's content, never escape from being the objects of never-ending resentment?[9]

We have seen, then, that there are a variety of arguments for and against transhumanism. It will be clear that I am not in favour of the radical or the less extreme versions. It seems clear to me at least that the project is an undesirable utopianism. We have enough problems with the human nature we struggle with, let alone another nature that we neither control nor understand anywhere near as fully. At TH's heart, it seems to me, is a view of technology at the mercy of scientists generally (or in the case of athletic powers, sports 'medics'), which is simply a case of Prometheanism. This charge is often labelled against genetic and other technologists without proper explanation. And it strikes me that the charge is not properly understood. In order to move beyond mere slogans or name-calling, then, I shall offer two contrasting lenses through which these claims may be viewed by returning to the roots of the Promethean myth itself.

6. Whose Prometheus: Hesiod or Aeschylus?

In order to understand the charge of Prometheanism one might begin by asking 'What is the myth of Prometheus?' I think the better question is 'whose myth of Prometheus should we concern ourselves with?' I take my cue from Conacher's (1980) account and also from Kerenyi's (1963), though I do not attempt fully to do justice to their accounts here.[10] I merely use them for my own purpose of providing lenses to view the unrestrained enhancement ideology of TH which, it seems to me, can find an easy footing in the unreflective pools of sports medicine and sports sciences more generally.

First, let us say that there is no single Greek account of Prometheus's deeds. There are at least two sources and even among these sources there are variations. The two sources, in chronology, are Hesiod and Aeschylus. In Hesiod there are two accounts: *Theogony* and *Works and Days*. And the only full text from Aeschylus is *Prometheus Bound*, though we know it to be part of a trilogy (with *Prometheus Unbound* and *Prometheus the Firebringer*).

Theogony is Hesiod's account of the beginning of the world. The Titans (giants) challenged Zeus and the Olympian Gods for the supremacy of the world. *Works and Days* is said to be a similar account, but one that celebrates the ideas that labour is the universal lot of mankind but that those willing so to do can get by. This is important to appreciate in order to evaluate the act for which Prometheus became (in)famous. Prometheus, acting against his fellow Titans, sided with Zeus and his cunning aided Zeus's victory over the Olympian Gods. In consequence he was honoured by Zeus and seems to have some kind of dual nature: both God and mortal. Sometimes the two are simplistically dichotomised: Zeus as power, Prometheus as cunning reason or intellect (Conacher 1980).

Prometheus is said to have stolen fire and to have cheated the gods out of their proper share of a sacrifice. Which came first is not always clear as there are different interpretations. But both acts, according to Kerenyi, evidence the claim that Prometheus is of deficient character. He writes:

> Prometheus, founder of the sacrifice, was a cheat and a thief: those traits are at the bottom of all the stories that deal with him. The meaning of his strange sacrifice in which the gods were cheated out of the tasty morsels is simply this: that the sacrifice offered up by men is a sacrifice of foolhardy thieves, stealers of the divinity round about them – for the world of nature that surrounds them is divine – whose temerity brings immeasurable and unforeseen misfortune upon them. (Kerenyi 1980, xxii)

A little amplification is in order. Both Prometheus (often translated as 'foresight') and his somewhat bungling brother Epimetheus (sometimes translated as 'aftersight') set out on Zeus's orders to fashion creatures to populate the earth. Lacking wisdom (or 'foresight') Epimetheus fails to consider what qualities are necessary as he goes about making the 'animal kingdom'. Prometheus fashions mortals in the vision of the gods. Epimetheus, having used all his gifts from Zeus, has failed to clothe them and Prometheus watches pitifully as they shiver in the cold nights. It is here that, rebelling against Zeus's authority, Prometheus sides with mankind, and steals fire – hidden in a fennel stalk. The mortals are thus warmed.

In order to appease and honour Zeus, Prometheus reveals his disrespectful cunning. He offers him an ox. In one half he hides the bones with a rich layering of fat which appears on the surface to be the greater and more desirable share. Under the entrails of the animal he hides in the other skin all the good meat. Zeus, apparently understanding the deception as part of the unchanging fate of mankind, accepts the lesser share.

By way of punishing Prometheus and all mortals, Zeus withheld fire from mortals.[11] The hubris of Prometheus in particular, though, is captured by his punishment: he is to be chained to a tree on Mount Caucasus where an eagle will eat at his liver all day only for it to be replenished over night for the cycle of suffering and humiliation to continue the next day, and so on.

In Aeschylus we get a different interpretation of events, one that is at once more sympathetic to Prometheus. First, a more optimistic conception of 'human initiative' (Conacher 1980, 13). A further aspect of this is the fact that hope is hidden from men in Hesiod ('fortunately', it is said in Hesiod, or rather 'for their sakes') whereas in Aeschylus it is one of the gifts from Prometheus. As Conacher puts it:

> To put the point in the broadest possible terms, the Hesiodic Prometheus, by his deceptions and frustrations of Zeus in his relations with man, is presented (however 'artificially') as the indirect cause of all man's woes; the Aeschylean Prometheus, on the other hand, by his interventions on behalf of man, is presented as the saviour of mankind, without whom man would have ceased to exist and with whose help he progresses from mere subsistence to a state of civilization. (Conacher 1980, 13)

Aeschylus does this by suppressing the sacrifice deception and transforms the fire-stealing act as one of daring rather than hubris. For without the deception there is no occasion for the withholding of fire, which is the consequent punishment. For fire is seen not merely as the warmth that forestalls the chill of the night but – more importantly – as the precondition of craft, trade, even civilization. But what has all this got to do with tranhsumanism generally, and sports medicine more specifically?

7. A Moral Topography for Sports Medicine

In the rise of psychiatry, much was made of the scientism that bedevilled the then emerging profession. Disputes raged as to whether there could be such a thing as mental illness (akin to physical illness) or whether this constituted the imposition of normative patterns of thought and action by state powers. The more pharmacologically inclined argued that mental illness did indeed exist but that its basis was chemical, not political. Others took it to be a case of the medicalisation of everyday life. In all of this Thomas Szasz was (and still remains) a trenchant critic. Like Kass, Szasz has been charged with providing powerful polemic more than patient argument. Notwithstanding this, he once crafted the memorable, remark that 'Formerly, when religion was strong and science weak, men mistook magic for medicine; now, when science is strong and religion weak, men mistake medicine for magic' (Szasz 1973, 115).

This juxtaposition of religion, magic and science is a troublesome one for the public no less than for gullible and overcommitted athletes who appear to lack any kind of moral framework within which to evaluate their Herculean efforts. The main concern which TH raises for sports is the following, rather general, concern: 'How are we to evaluate the enhancement agenda?' It is clear that there are strong advocates such as Miah who want to extend autonomous choice by athletes in ways that may easily open the door for unprincipled biomedical and sports scientists. Equally clearly there will be traditionalists, myself included, who find the unfettered use of technology to augment human nature utterly repellent.

One way forward is to establish better spaces of dialogue between opposing camps in order to establish what Taylor (1991) calls 'moral topography'. I take this to be a loose application of what he had in mind in his articulation of the moral sources of modern identity. Moral topography in sports medicine might be about drawing out the conceptual relief and the natural and artificial aspects of the work of scientists therein. I use moral topography as a metaphor for teasing out what I take to be the 'traditional' (natural?) work of medicine in the relief of suffering and the more recent (and artificial) goal of performance enhancement or the augmentation of natural abilities as opposed to the traditional therapeutic role of medicine. This may help develop critical but informed attitudes to, for example, the new genetic technologies which are likely to invade elite sports over the next decade and which threaten to make arcane the worries over steroids, EPO or human growth hormone.

But in contrast to Miah (2004), and to Jonas (1974) and Kass (2002) before him, the new biology and biotechnology or indeed the new genetics need not require us to rethink a new ethics *ab initio*. The sources for the evaluation of medical and sports technology were revealed long ago in the ancient Greek writings of Plato. The historian of medicine Edelstein (1967) notes the ancient Greek philosopher's task of undermining the glorification of the body. And building upon his insight McKenny (1997) noted Plato's observations, considering the education of the 'Guardians' so that medicine may serve rather than hinder or dominate our moral projects. In this vein we too should ask: How much attention should we devote to our bodies in the effort to optimise our capacities? How much control should we allow physicians to exercise over our bodies? What ends should determine what counts as a sufficiently healthy body? What limits should we observe in our efforts to improve our bodily performance and remove causes of suffering?

Elite sportsmen and women, their coaches, sports national governing bodies and even sports promoters and institutions such as the IOC, the IAAF and FIFA, all have an interest in surpassing limits. Athletes are deemed to have failed if they do not 'peak' at big events, breaking their own personal best times, heights or distances. World records must tumble at every event, it seems. At this macro-level, enhanced performances are wrapped up in celebratory spectacles primarily to sell media and marketing packages. And the circus rolls on to the next event, the next town. This denial of the necessity of limits in nature by some, the desire to remove or delay their onset in the shape of disease or burnout-syndrome and to control these human-limiting factors by the unfettered use of biotechnology is something that should concern us all in sports. I submit that philosophers of both sport and medicine begin to press such questions home in the public spaces of the media as well as the gymnasium and the university so that sports do not become the vanguard of Hesiod's Promethean project.[12]

NOTES

1.   The best known advocate for which is Andy Miah 2004.
2.   For an example of such conceptual inflation see Brülde 2001.
3.   See for example Shilling 2005.

4. The conflation of terms goes worse than this. In my view a significant portion of what is called 'sports medicine' is not medicine at all, but more commonly sports science or sports technology. See Edwards and McNamee 2006.
5. See http://en.wikipedia.org/wiki/Biotechnology, accessed 6 June 2006.
6. For a debate on the pros and cons of hypoxic chambers as (il)licit uses of sports medicine see Spriggs 2005 and the collected responses by Fricker 2005 Tamburrini 2005 and Tännsjö 2005 which were published recently in the *Journal of Medical Ethics*.
7. For a fuller account of the nature(s) of TH see McNamee and Edwards 2006.
8. The clearest expositor is Nick Boström, See his 'Transhumanist values' (2005b). See also Boström 2005a, and contrast with the outline of one of the movement's founding fathers Max More (More 1996; 2005). For a more detailed summary of the purported features of TH see McNamee and Edwards 2005.
9. As Rollin 2003 remarked of those who in the future might develop, and retain the secrets of, extreme longevity.
10. A short summary of the two accounts, though with no comparison or contrast, can be found in Price and Kearns 2004, 453.
11. There is some ambiguity as to whether mortals had fire before. Conacher (1980, 12) is in no doubt that Prometheus stole it back for them, which entails their prior possession of it. I set to one side here Hesiod's misogynistic account of the first punishment intended for Prometheus, where Zeus has Hephaestus fashion woman from fire (namely Pandora) whose jar (and not 'box' as is commonly thought) contains all the portents for the suffering of mankind.
12. I am grateful to Fritz-Gregor Herrman for his insight and guidance regarding the myths of Prometheus. I am especially grateful to my colleague Steve Edwards, with whom I have collaborated closely on issues regarding both transhumanism – especially in the light of 'slippery slope' arguments – (McNamee and Edwards 2006) and also regarding the conceptual relations between medicine and sports medicine (Edwards and McNamee 2006). This essay is an offshoot from those discussions and conferences which was previously presented at a conference in Prague and which was published in an earlier form in Slovenian (McNamee 2005) and has been significantly revised.

REFERENCES

BACON, F. 2000. *Novum Organon,* edited by L. Jardine and M. Silverthorne. Cambridge: Cambridge University Press.

BORGMANN, A. 1984. *Technology and the Character of Everyday Life.* Chicago: University of Chicago Press.

BOSTRÖM, N. 2004. Human genetic enhancements: A transhumanist perspective. *The Journal of Value Inquiry* 37 (4): 493 – 506.

———. 2005a. The fable of the dragon tyrant. *Journal of Medical Ethics* 31: 231 – 7.

———. 2005b. Transhumanist values, available at http://www.nickBoström.com/ethics/values.html, accessed 19 May 2005.

BRÜLDE, B. 2001. The goals of medicine: towards a unified theory. *Health Care Analysis* 9: 1 – 13.

CASSELL, E. 2004. *The Nature of Suffering.* 2nd edn. Oxford: Oxford University Press.

CONACHER, D.J. 1980. *Aeschylus' Prometheus Bound.* Toronto: University of Toronto Press.

DESAUER, F. 1927. *Philosophie der Technik.* Bonn: Verlag.

DESCARTES, R. 2003. *Discourse on method and related writings* (translated by Desmond M. Clarke). London: Penguin.

EDELSTEIN, L. 1967. *Ancient Medicine*, edited by O. Temkin and L. Temkin. Baltimore, MD: Johns Hopkins University Press.

EDWARDS, S.D. and M.J. MCNAMEE. 2006. Why sports medicine is *not* medicine. *Health Care Analysis* 2006 (14): 103–9.

ELLUL, J. 1965. *The Technological Society,* trans. J. Wilkinson. London: Cape.

FOUCAULT, M. 1988. *Technologies of the Self*, edited by L.H. Martin, H. Gutman, and P.H. Hutton, Amherst, MA: University of Massachusetts Press.

FRICKER, P. 2005. Hypoxic air machines: Commentary. *Journal of Medical Ethics* 31: 115.

HABERMAS, J. 1968. *Knowledge and Human Interests*. Cambridge: Polity (repr. 1986).

———. 2003. *The Future of Human Nature*. Cambridge: Polity.

HEIDEGGER, M. 1977. *The Question Concerning Technology and Other Essays,* trans. W. Lovitt. San Francisco, CA: Harper Row.

HICKMAN, L.A. 2001. *Philosophical Tools for Technological Culture: Putting Pragmatism to Work.* Bloomington, IN: Indiana University Press.

JONAS, H. 1974. *Philosophical Essays: From Ancient Creed to Technological Man.* Chicago: University of Chicago Press.

KASS, L. 2002. *Life, Liberty and the Defense of Dignity*. San Francisco, CA: Encounter Books.

KAPP, F. 1877. *Grundlinien einer Philosophie der Technik*. Braunshcweig: Westermann.

KERENYI, C. 1963. *Prometheus*. Princeton, NJ. Princeton University Press.

LEE, K. 2003. *Philosophy and Revolutions in Genetics*. London: Palgrave.

LEWIS, C.S. 1943. *The Abolition of Man*. Oxford: Oxford University Press.

MCKENNY, G.P. 1997. *To Relieve the Human Condition*. Brockport, NY: SUNY Press.

MCNAMEE, M.J. 2005. Transhumanizem in moralna topografija sportne medicine ['transhumanism and the moral topography of sports medicine', in Slovenian]. *Borec* 57: 626–9.

MCNAMEE, M.J. and S.D. EDWARDS. 2006. Transhumanism, medical technology, and slippery slopes. *Journal of Medical Ethics* 32: 513–18.

MARCUSE, H. 1964. *One Dimensional Man*. Boston, MA: Beacon Press.

MIAH, A. 2004. *Genetically Modified Athletes*. London: Routledge.

MITCHAM, C. 1979. Philosophy and the history of technology. In *The History and Philosophy of Technology*, edited by G. Bugliarello and D.B. Doner. London: University of Illinois Press.

———. 1995. Philosophy and technology. In *Encyclopedia of bioethics*, edited by W.T. Reich. London: Simon and Schuster: 2477–84.

MORE, M. 1996. Transhumanism: Towards a futurist philosophy, available at http://www.maxmore.com/transhum.htm, accessed 20 July 2005.

———. 2005. Available at http://www.mactonnies.com/trans.html, accessed 13 July 2005.

NYE, D.E. 2006. *Technology Matters*. London: MIT Press.

ORTEGA Y GASSET, J. 1941. "Man the technician" in *Towards a philosophy of history*. New York: Norton.

PARENS, E. 1995. The goodness of fragility: On the prospects of genetic technologies aimed at the enhancement of human capacities. *Kennedy Institute of Ethics Journal* 5 (2): 131–43.

PORTER, R. 2002. *Blood and guts: A short history of medicine*. London: Penguin.

PRICE, S. AND E. KEARNS. 2004. *Oxford Dictionary of Classical Myth and Religion*. Oxford: Oxford University Press.

ROLLIN, B. 2003. Telos, value and genetic engineering. In *Is Human Nature Obsolete?* edited by H.W. Baillie and T.K. Casey. Cambridge, MA: MIT Press, 317–26.

SANDBERG, A. 2001. Morphological freedom – why we not just want it but need it. Paper presented to TransVision 2001 conference, Berlin, available at http://www.nada.kth.se/~asa/Texts/MorphologicalFreedom.htm, accessed 5 Oct. 2005.

SHILLING, C. 2005. *The Body in Culture, Technology and Society.* London: Sage.

SPRIGGS, M. 2005. Hypoxic air machines: Performance enhancement through effective training – or cheating? *Journal of Medical Ethics* 31: 112–13.

SZASZ, T. 1973. *The Second Sin.* London: Routledge.

TAMBURRINI, C. 2005. Hypoxic air machines: Commentary. *Journal of Medical Ethics* 31: 114.

TANNSJÖ, T. 2005. Hypoxic air machines: Commentary. *Journal of Medical Ethics* 31: 112–13.

TAYLOR, C. 1991. *Sources of the Self.* Cambridge: Cambridge University Press.

UNITED NATIONS CONVENTION ON BIOLOGICAL DIVERSITY. 1992. Available at http://en.wikipedia.org/wiki/Convention_on_Biological_Diversity, accessed 10 June 2006.

WORLD TRANSHUMANIST ASSOCIATION. Available at http://www.transhumanism.org/index.php/WTA/index/, accessed 7 April 2006.

'HUMAN-NESS', 'DEHUMANISATION' AND PERFORMANCE ENHANCEMENT

Leon Culbertson

This paper focuses on the claim by Schneider and Butcher (2000) that it makes little sense to criticise the use of performance-enhancing drugs as 'dehumanising' (as, for example, Hoberman does (1992)) because we are unable to give a satisfactory account of what it is to be human. Schneider and Butcher (2000, 196) put this as follows: 'The dehumanisation argument is interesting but incomplete. It is incomplete because we do not have an agreed-upon conception of what it is to be human. Without this it is difficult to see why some practices should count as dehumanising.' The paper begins by considering J.L. Austin's (1962) treatment of the word 'real'. By transposing ideas from Austin to the terms 'dehumanise' and 'human' I argue that (a) In the pair 'dehumanise' and 'human', the term 'dehumanise' is dominant; (b) We cannot understand 'dehumanise' and 'human' independently of either the context of their use or the contrast that is drawn in their use; (c) Either one of these is sufficient to understand the terms; (d) 'Dehumanise', 'human' and their cognates are not univocal; we can have no recourse to exceptionless accounts of the meaning of such terms. The importance of context is developed further by consideration of an example from the work of Charles Travis (2005), and the issue of exceptionless accounts of the meaning of words is addressed through an application of Gordon Baker's (2004) characterisation of Wittgenstein's uses of the term 'metaphysical' to Miah's (2004) treatment of human-ness. I argue that Miah's conception of human-ness exhibits all the forms of metaphysical use of terms (in this case the term 'human') outlined by Baker (2004). The article attempts to clarify some objections to the use of performance-enhancing drugs and the prospect of genetic modification of athletes by sketching an overview of possible concrete uses of 'dehumanise'. The focus of the paper, however, is on 'making sense of what we (are inclined to) say ... [rather than] making explicit what underlies what we say' (McFee, 1993/4, 115).

Resumen

Este artículo se centra en la afirmación de Schenider y Butcher (2000) de que tiene poco sentido el criticar el uso de drogas que mejoren el rendimiento físico como "deshumanizantes" (como por ejemplo hace Hoberman (1992)) ya que no somos capaces de dar una idea satisfactoria sobre lo que es un ser humano. Schneider y Butcher (2000, 196) lo ponen de la siguiente manera: 'El argumento de la deshumanización es interesante pero incompleto. Es incompleto porque no hay un acuerdo sobre la concepción de lo que es un ser humano. Sin esto es dificil el ver como cierttas prácticas pueden ser tomadas en cuenta como deshumanizantes'.

El artículo empieza con una consideración de como J.L. Austin manejó la palabra 'real'. Por medio de una trasposición de las ideas de Austin a los términos 'deshumanizar' y 'humano' argumento que: (a) en la pareja 'deshumanizar' y 'humano', el término 'deshumanizar' es dominante. (b) No podemos entender 'deshumanizar' y 'humano' independientemente bien del contexto de su uso, bien del contraste que se abstrae de su uso. (c) Cualquiera de los dos es suficiente para entender los términos. (d) "deshumanizar', 'humano' y sus cognados no son unívocos; no podemos recurrir a explicaciones sin excepciones sobre el significado de tales términos.

La importancia del contexto es desarrollada aún más por medio de la consideración de un ejemplo de la obra de Charles Tracis (2005), y el tema de explicaciones sin excepciones del significado de las palabras se trata por medio de una aplicación de la caracterización que Gordon Baker (2004), quien por medio de Wittgenstein y sus usos del término 'metafísico', aplica al tratamiento que Miah (2004) da al human-ismo. Argumento que la concepción de Miah de human-ismo presenta todas las formas del uso metafísico de los términos (en este caso el término 'humano') tal y como ha sido perfilado por Baker (2004).

El artículo intenta aclarar algunas objeciones al uso de drogas que mejoran el rendimiento físico y el prospecto de la modificación genética de los atletas por medio del bosquejo de una visión general de los posibles usos concretos de 'deshumanizar'. El foco del artículo, sin embargo es el 'dar sentido a lo que decimos (o tendemos a decir)...[en vez de] ...hacer explícito lo que hay por debajo de lo que decimos' (McFee, 1993/4, 115).

Zusammenfassung

Dieser Aufsatz nimmt die Behauptung von Schneider und Butcher (2000) in den Blick, in der sie äußern, dass es wenig Sinn mache, die Einnahme leitungssteigernder Mittel als ,entmenschlichend' zu klassifizieren (wie es beispielsweise Hoberman (1992) tat), da wir nicht in der Lage seien eine zufriedenstellende Aussage darüber zu machen, was es denn eigentlich bedeute Mensch zu sein? Ohne diese Grundlage sei es schwierig zu verstehen, warum einige Praktiken als ,entmens-chlichend' betrachtet werden sollten.

Den Anfang dieses Artikels bilden Überlegungen zu J. L. Austins (1962) Verwendung des Begriffs ,wirklich'. Die Anwendung von Austins Gedanken auf die Begriffe ,entmenschlichen' und ,menschlich' führt zu folgenden Behauptungen: (a) Im Begriffspaar ,entmenschlichen' und ,menschlich', dominiert der Begriff ,entmenschlichen'. (b) Es ist unmöglich ein Verständnis der Begriffe ,entmenschlichen' und ,menschlich' unabhängig vom Kontext ihrer Verwendung zu entwickeln, oder unhabhängig vom Gegensatz der durch ihre Verwendung dargestellt werden soll. (c) Lediglich einer der vorgenannten Aspekte ist zum näheren Verständnis der Begriffe ausreichend. (d) Die Begriffe ,entmenschlichen', ,menschlich' sowie deren Bergiffsverwandte sind nicht eindeutig; wir können also nicht auf eine zweifelsfreie Bedeutungszuschreibung dieser Worte zurückgreifen.

Mit Hilfe der Arbeit von Charles Travis (2005) wird die Wichtigkeit des Kontextes näher ausgeführt. Des Weiteren wird durch die Anwendung von Gordon Bakers (2004) Charakterisierung von Wittgensteins Verwendung des Begriffs ,metaphysisch' auf Miah (2004), insbesondere Miahs Gebrauch des Begriffs human-ness (=menschl. Natur/menschl. Lebewesen) das Problem der Eindeutigkeit/Ausnahmslosigkeit angesprochen. Meines Erachtens weist Miahs Begriffsbildung human-ness alle Formen eines metaphysischen Sprachgebrauchs auf (in diesem Fall der Begriff ,menschlich') wie sie von Baker (2004) umschrieben wurden.

Dieser Artikel versucht die Einwände gegen den Gebrauch leistungssteigernder Substanzen, sowie die zu erwartende genetische Veränderung von Sporltern, durch die Skizzierung möglicher Konkretisierungen des Begriffs ‚entmenschlichen', zu schärfen. Der Schwerpunkt dieses Textes liegt jedoch eher in der ‚Bedeutungsbestimmung dessen was wir sagen (zu sagen beabsichtigen)… [als]… der Explizierung dessen was unserem Gesagtem zugrunde liegt.' (McFee, 1993/4, 115).

摘要

本文是針對 Schneider 與 Butcher (2000) 的主張來做一討論。他們的主張認為：用一種 "去人性化"（dehumanizing）的觀點去批判會增進運動表現的藥物使用方法並不具有太大的意義（就如 Hoberman (1992) 所說的）。因為我們不能夠給出一個令人滿足的說法來解釋何謂人性。Schneider 與 Butcher (2000, 196) 提到以下觀點："去人性化的主張是有趣的，但不夠完整。它不夠完整是因為我們並不具備一個大家所同意之人性概念。因為無此一共識，我們很難去了解為何一些活動就應該視為去人性化。"

本文一開始考慮到 J. L. Austin (1962) 對 "real" 這個字的處理。藉由 Austin 對 "去人性"（dehumanize）與 "人性"（human）互調出來所討論出的結果，我主張：(a) 在 "去人性" 與 "人性" 這一對字詞中，"去人性" 扮演主宰的角色. (b) 假設不考慮到情境，以及兩者對照之使用，我們是無法了解 "去人性" 與 "人性" 兩者之意涵 (c) 但只要有其中一項出現，我們就可以了解其兩者之意涵。(d) "去人性"、"人性" 及其同類詞語並不是單義的；我們不能依賴無例外的字義說法存在。

更進一步地，有關情境的重要文獻，可以考慮到 Charles Travis (2005) 的主張，以及 Gordon Baker (2004) 提到有關字義的無例外說法的課題應用：將維根斯坦 (Wittgenstein) 對 "形上學上"（metaphysical）術語的描述應用至 Miah (2004) 對人性（human-ness）的處理。我認為 Miah 的 human-ness（人性）概念是藉由 Baker (2004) 所勾勒的思想展現出形上學上字義的所有使用形式（在此例為 'human' 這個字）。

本文藉著探討一些 "去人性" 這個詞的可能具體使用方式來澄清一些對增進運動表現藥物使用上的反對論點，以及了解到基因改造下的運動員之前景。不過，本文主要在於處理 "我們所（想要）說的話是否有道理…而非將一些字面下的意義做一明確的表達"（McFee, 1993/4, 115）。

This article aims to address what I take to be two misconceptions about performance enhancement in sports ethics and sports medicine. First, the view that the moral evaluation of performance enhancement requires a clear idea of what it is to be human (Miah 2004, 65 and 71); and second, the related view that one cannot claim that methods of performance enhancement are 'dehumanising' because, as Schneider and Butcher (2000, 196) put it:

'The dehumanisation argument is interesting but incomplete. It is incomplete because we do not have an agreed-upon conception of what it is to be human. Without this it is difficult to see why some practices should count as dehumanising.'

Baker and Hacker (1984, 12) describe part of their strategy in *Language, Sense and Nonsense* as 'focus[ing] on the logically prior questions of the intelligibility and purpose of salient theses'. This allows them to 'by-pass controversies about the truth or falsity of various doctrines in theories of meaning'. This strategy is adopted as a result of a commitment to the view that 'it is a mistake in addressing theories of meaning to rush headlong into attempts at testing their truth or falsity.' This approach is useful in addressing the misconceptions targeted by this article. First, could there be such a thing as 'an agreed-upon conception of what it is to be human'? Second, is there *necessarily* a connection between 'dehumanise' and 'human-ness'? Third, does the prefix 'de-' *always* function in the same way in 'dehumanise' as it does in, for example, 'decapitate'? Fourth, could a human being ever not be, or be less, human? In one sense of the word 'human' (i.e. as members of *homo sapiens*) we surely *cannot* be anything *other* than human.[1] If we exist *at all* (even as a dead body), we exist as members of *homo sapiens*. Yet, clearly this is not the *relevant sense* of 'human' in this case. However, human-ness does not appear to admit of degrees. Would we not be treating existence as a predicate if we were to regard human-ness as something we could have to varying degrees? Perhaps we can be not, or less, human if we take human-ness to be a culturally relative social construct; perhaps we should view human-ness as in some way connected to morality. But we *do* have generally accepted conceptions of human-ness in this sense. Within cultures there are dominant notions of morality, regardless of how many people allow those notions to inform their actions. Does this not mean that Schneider and Butcher's (2000) point collapses? Fifth, are 'dehumanise' and 'human-ness' *each* univocal? And sixth, does 'human-ness' refer to a 'thing'? 'Thing' here indicates an assumption that there is something hidden which must be uncovered – perhaps a univocal meaning, perhaps a more concrete 'thing', such as a human essence as some form of behaviour, mental process, neurological hardware, capacity etc. If 'human-ness' does refer to a 'thing', does 'dehumanise' refer to a lack of that 'thing'? The backdrop to the sixth question(s) is referential theories of meaning, which hold that *all* words (as opposed to just *some* words) refer to something, sometimes only abstract entities, and that the meaning of words is the thing that they refer to.

I have set a great many hares running here and will, in time, catch up with each of them. By then, however, it will be apparent that many of these questions are ill-conceived. Reaching an awareness of this is a valuable step in its own right. I argue here that 'human-ness' is what Austin (1962, 70) called 'a *trouser-word*'.[2] In other words, it is the negative form ('dehumanise') rather than the affirmative form ('human-ness') that is dominant, or 'wears the trousers'.[3] This means that we understand concrete uses of 'dehumanise' either from the context or the contrast that is drawn in each particular case. I also argue that attempts to provide exceptionless accounts of the meaning of 'dehumanise', 'human-ness' and their cognates leads to the kind of problems Wittgenstein was trying to help us to avoid when he pointed out that 'what *we* do is to bring words back from their metaphysical to their everyday use' (*PI*, §116).[4] The article attempts to show that an understanding of human-ness cannot possibly be the basis of moral evaluations of performance enhancement. Nor is it possible to sustain the position outlined by Schneider and Butcher (2000, 196). This will be done by sketching an overview of possible concrete uses of 'dehumanise', 'human' and their cognates. The focus of the paper, however, is on 'making sense of what we (are inclined to) say...[rather than] making explicit what *underlies* what we say' (McFee 1993/4, 115).

I will begin by outlining the notion of a 'trouser-word' through consideration of J.L. Austin's discussion of the word 'real'. Following this I will argue that 'human-ness' is a trouser-word and then elaborate two further points which emerge in Austin's discussion of 'real': first, Austin's criticism of exceptionless accounts of the meaning of words will be developed further through consideration of Wittgenstein's remarks on metaphysical/everyday use. Second, the relevance of context will be explored through consideration of examples from the work of Charles Travis. These discussions will prepare the ground for some remarks on the need for occasion-sensitivity and the role of ostensive, rather than verbal, definitions of 'dehumanise', 'human-ness' and their cognates.

Austin on 'Real'

Austin makes four points about the word 'real'. Of these, three are relevant in relation to 'dehumanise' and 'human'.[5]

1. *'Real' is substantive-hungry.* He (Austin 1962, 68) asks us to consider the following two pairs of sentences:

> 'These diamonds are real'; 'These are real diamonds'.
> 'These diamonds are pink'; 'These are pink diamonds'.

Austin's point is that we can say that something is *pink* without knowing what that thing *is*, or without making any reference to the *thing itself*. However, we cannot do this with 'real'. This is because something 'may be both a real *x* and not a real *y*' (Austin 1962, 69). In the case of uses of 'real', we must be able to answer the question 'A real *what*?' (ibid.).[6] 'Human' is also substantive-hungry in so far as we cannot say that someone is acting in a proper human manner (for example as a moral agent acting in the way we would expect such agents to act) without knowing *what* the person's actions are.

Austin stresses that it is not always appropriate to ask whether something is real. The question 'Is it real or not?' is only appropriate if there could possibly be an alternative to what appears to be the case. Only when 'suspicion assails us', when we think that things 'may not be what they seem' (Austin 1962, 69), is it appropriate to raise the question of the reality of an entity or phenomenon.

Equally, it is not always appropriate to ask about human-ness; there must first be some apparent alternative. This leads directly to Austin's second point:

2. *'Real' is a trouser-word.* Austin's point here is that while in many cases we correctly treat the affirmative use of a term as the basic use and allow it to determine what constitutes appropriate use of the negative form of the word, it is not correct to use *all* words which have affirmative and negative forms in this way. Austin points out that in the case of 'real', 'it is the *negative* use that wears the trousers.[7] That is, a definite sense attaches to the assertion that something is real – a real such-and-such – only in the light of a specific way in which it might be, or might have been, *not* real' (Austin 1962, 70). He continues:

> 'A real duck' differs from the simple 'a duck' only in that it is used to exclude various ways of being not a real duck – but a dummy, a toy, a picture, a decoy, &c.; and moreover I

don't know *just* how to take the assertion that it is a real duck unless I know *just* what, on that particular occasion, the speaker has in mind to exclude. This, of course, is why the attempt to find a characteristic common to all things that are or could be called 'real' is doomed to failure;[8] the function of 'real' is not to contribute positively to the characterization of anything, but to exclude possible ways of being *not* real – and these ways are both numerous for particular kinds of things, and liable to be quite different for things of different kinds. (Austin 1962, 70)

Austin makes the point that the fact that there is an identity to the 'general function' of 'real' while it also has an 'immense diversity in [its] specific applications' (Austin 1962, 71) means that it is, rather confusingly, neither univocal nor ambiguous.

There are a number of important points which can be drawn from this in relation to 'human'. First, with 'human' it is the negative rather than the affirmative use which is dominant. So we can only make sense of talk of human-ness by reference to particular ways that *something* might be *dehumanising*, or *someone* might be *dehumanised*. Second, this means that talk of human-ness is context-specific; I cannot understand reference to human-ness without knowing what ways in which something might be dehumanising (or someone dehumanised) the speaker has in mind in drawing the contrast in *this* particular context. Consequently, third, 'human', 'dehumanise' and their cognates are *not* univocal. The function of 'human-ness' is to exclude possible ways of being not human, and there are a range of possible ways that one might be taken to be not human (as a moral agent), or one's actions to be 'dehumanising'.

Unlike 'real', there is no identity to the general function of 'human'; it can refer to membership of *homo sapiens*, or to moral agency. Like 'real', however, there is great diversity in the specific applications of 'human-ness' and 'dehumanise'. As a consequence, both terms and their cognates are not univocal but, unlike 'real', they are *potentially* ambiguous in the sense that they do have more than one meaning.[9]

3. *'Real' is a dimension-word.* The point Austin wishes to make here is that 'real' is the most general term in a family of words serving the same function. As the words in that family become more specific they give a clearer indication of what is being excluded.[10] This is also true of 'human'; we can identify collections of words on both the affirmative and the negative side which vary in their specificity, and of which 'human' and 'dehumanise' or 'inhuman' are the most general terms in each group. For example, on the affirmative side we might include 'human', 'person', 'agent', 'moral agent', 'natural', 'authentic', 'cultured', 'civilised', 'sensitive' and 'sympathetic'. On the negative side we might include 'dehumanise', 'inhuman', 'automaton', 'unnatural', 'animal', 'inauthentic', 'uncultured', 'uncivilised', 'desensitised' and 'unsympathetic'. It might also be appropriate to consider 'good' and 'bad' as in some way being connected to these groups of words.

An important point here is that on the affirmative side the various words serve to exclude possible ways of being *not* human, yet if the more general term of 'human' is used in any particular case it is still possible to understand its use by reference to the context. So we have two ways of understanding the use of 'human' and 'dehumanise'; we can look at the context, or we can consider the contrast that is being drawn. While we may not be able to do both in every case, it will always be possible to do one of the two and that is sufficient to understand the use of the term.

In summary, key points to draw from this discussion of Austin on 'real' are: (a) In the pair 'dehumanise' and 'human', the term 'dehumanise' is dominant. (b) We cannot understand 'dehumanise' and 'human' independently of either the context of their use *or* the contrast that is drawn in their use. (c) Either one of these is sufficient to understand the terms. (d) We can have no recourse to exceptionless accounts of the meaning of 'dehumanise' and 'human'; these terms and their cognates are *not* univocal. The final point here can be elaborated by considering G.P. Baker's reading of Wittgenstein's distinction between metaphysical and everyday use. Having highlighted the implications of that work, I will develop points (b) – (d) above by making a case for occasion-sensitivity in attempting to understand the use of 'dehumanise', 'human' and their cognates.

Wittgenstein on Metaphysical/Everyday Use

Austin (1962, 68) argued that 'real' is 'substantive-hungry' and that 'the attempt to find a characteristic common to all things that are or could be called 'real' is doomed to failure' (Austin 1962, 70). It has been argued here that both these points apply to 'human' and 'dehumanise'. Wittgenstein identifies the problem that substantives cause:

> The questions 'What is length?', 'What is meaning?', 'What is the number one?' etc., produce in us a mental cramp. We feel that we can't point to anything in reply to them and yet ought to point to something. (We are up against one of the great sources of philosophical bewilderment: a substantive makes us look for a thing that corresponds to it.) (*BB*: 1).

This is the terrain of the logically prior question raised above: does 'human-ness' refer to a 'thing'? And if it does, does 'dehumanise' refer to a lack of that 'thing'? Wittgenstein points out that 'studying the grammar of the expression "explanation of meaning" will teach you something about the grammar of the word "meaning" and will cure you of the temptation to look about you *for some object* which you might call "the meaning"' (my italics) (*BB*: 1). The same point applies to 'human' and 'dehumanise'; there is *nothing* to point *to* in these cases and this is shown by consideration of the grammar of expressions containing those terms.[11]

A common interpretation (perhaps even the 'standard' interpretation) of Wittgenstein's 'metaphysical'/'everyday' distinction is that 'everyday' is the dominant term. Baker (2004) looks at a range of examples of Wittgenstein's use of 'metaphysical' and its cognates. From this he identifies a number of patterns that emerge (there is no single pattern). The conclusion that Baker reaches is that

> Within the corpus of Wittgenstein's texts, the term 'metaphysical' has a definite and quite traditional meaning: it belongs to a semantic field that includes 'necessary', 'essence', and 'nature'.... Granted that the phrases 'metaphysical use' and 'everyday use' are mutually exclusive, the term 'everyday' must be glossed as 'non-metaphysical'. Hence, in this pair, the term 'metaphysical' wears the trousers; and the term 'everyday' need *not* mean 'conforming with standard speech-practice'. (Baker 2004, 100)

The patterns of Wittgenstein's use of 'metaphysical' that are identified by Baker (2004) have an important bearing on the treatment of 'human' and 'dehumanise' and warrant an *apparent* scholarly digression.[12] Baker (2004) identifies four patterns to Wittgenstein's use of 'metaphysical':

1. '*Expressions of necessity and impossibility*, on statements that feature "must" and "cannot": non-scientific statements featuring such modal expressions are taken to be *overtly* metaphysical' (Baker 2004, 97).[13]
2. 'The use of words *without antitheses*:...Metaphysical propositions seem to be assertions of the greatest moment, formulating the very essence of things. At the same time, the impossibility of things' being otherwise opens the way to the recurrent criticism that metaphysical statements make applications of the key terms *redundant* and the assertions themselves empty' (Baker 2004, 98; also see *PI*, §131).[14] In these cases Wittgenstein is not referring to the use of words without negation, but rather assertions of necessity, essence or the nature of something which make it impossible for that thing to be otherwise. For example, in relation to human-ness, metaphysical uses in the sense Baker is referring to here are not uses of 'human' that deny the possibility of something being *not* human, but assertions about the nature of human-ness that preclude the possibility of human-ness being otherwise.
3. '*Non-scientific* statements having the *form* of *scientific* explanations (theories): formulations of essences often take the form of simple formulae giving definite answers to questions of the form "what is...?".' (Baker 2004, 98)

    For example, attempts to answer questions such as 'What is time?' (Waismann 1965, 172), 'What is length?', 'What is meaning?', 'What is the number one?' (*BB*, 1), or 'What is a proposition?' (*PI*, §92) are likely to produce metaphysical statements because the answer that is given is likely to be some form of exceptionless definition. The apparent similarity between such definitions and 'scientific truth[s]' (*BB*, 55), providing the kind of account which suggests that 'a stupendous discovery has been made' (*BB*, 23), is even more likely to confuse us than modal statements.[15]

    Baker (2004, 99) highlights the key point here by citing Wittgenstein's claim that 'The essential thing about metaphysics: that the difference between factual and conceptual investigations is not clear to it. A metaphysical question is always **in appearance** a factual one, although the problem is a conceptual one' (Baker's emphasis) (*RPP* I, §949; cf. *BB*, 35).[16] Baker (2004) rightly regards this as a major obstacle to acceptance of the correct way to resolve our philosophical perplexity – detailed consideration of how we use words.
4. 'Statements about word-use giving *explanations grounded in the natures* of things: for example, "it looks to us as if we were saying something about the **nature** of red in saying that the words 'Red exists' do not yield a sense" ([*PI*], §58). Likewise, in denying that a human *body can* have pain "it is as though we looked into the **nature** of pain and saw that it lies in its **nature** that a material object **can't** have it"' (*BB*, 73; Baker's emphasis) (Baker 2004, 99).

The importance of these distinctions becomes clear if we consider a prominent example of the treatment of 'human' and its cognates within the philosophy of sport, Miah's (2004) *Genetically Modified Athletes: Biomedical Ethics, Gene Doping and Sport*. Here we find many passages exhibiting a number of the features of metaphysical use outlined by Baker (2004). For example, Miah (2004, 65) claims that: 'The ethical limits of using genetics in sport *must* begin with a consideration of *what it means to be human*' (my emphasis). This is a non-scientific expression of necessity featuring 'must' (cf. Baker's (2004) first pattern of the use of 'metaphysical' and its cognates by Wittgenstein). When Miah (2004, 68) claims that 'Philosophical articulations of the human demonstrate a tendency to answer the question "*What is human?*" by contrasting it with other kinds of entity, such as animals, machines and automata' (my emphasis), he does not claim that there is anything wrong with the question 'What is human?' (including what is either poor grammar or a lack of quotation marks around 'human').[17] The question 'What is human?' calls for a non-scientific statement in the form of a scientific explanation; it requires a definite answer reached by the formulation of an essence of what it is to be human (cf. Baker's (2004) third pattern of the use of 'metaphysical' and its cognates by Wittgenstein).

Any doubt as to Miah's (2004) essentialism is removed by the following: 'I suggest that, in principle, Fukuyama is right;[18] *there is some Factor X* [i.e. a *human essence*] *that requires greater articulation*. Moreover, his approach to capture this within a discourse of human rights can serve as a starting point for *greater elaboration of humanness*' (Miah 2004, 71; my emphasis). Again the search for an essence is revealing of a metaphysical use of 'human' and its cognates (cf. Baker's (2004) third pattern of the use of 'metaphysical' and its cognates by Wittgenstein). There are also parallels between Baker's fourth use of 'metaphysical' and Miah's question '*How do humans differ from non-humans, or more simply, **what does it mean to be human**?*' (Miah 2004, 69; my emphasis). Here he is asking about the *nature* of human-ness in an attempt to clarify our *use* of the term 'human'.

Finally, Miah (2004, 65) cites both Schneider and Butcher (2000) and Loland (2000) in support of his own approach to human-ness, as holders of the view that '*defining the human* has a bearing upon what kinds of technology are acceptable for use in sport, arguing that sporting value is *inextricable* from being human' (my emphasis). The notion that we can/must *define* the human is a metaphysical use of 'human' in the third sense identified by Baker (2004) – a search for 'simple formulae giving definite answers to questions of the form "what is ...?"' (Baker 2004, 98). In addition, the claim that 'sporting value is *inextricable* from being human' (my italics) is a non-scientific expression of necessity akin to those featuring the modal term 'must' (cf. Baker's (2004) first pattern of the use of 'metaphysical' and its cognates by Wittgenstein).

The questions 'What is human?' and 'What does it mean to be human?', and the notions of a human essence and defining the human are all related to the second pattern of Wittgenstein's use of metaphysical and its cognates identified by Baker (2004) – the use of words without antitheses. The search for definiteness here is in pursuit of an account of what it is to be human that precludes the possibility of human-ness being otherwise.

Thus far, I have argued that in the pair 'dehumanise' and 'human-ness', 'dehumanise' is dominant. I have also argued that context and the contrasts drawn in the use of terms such as 'dehumanise' and 'human-ness' are central to our ability to understand those terms, and that it is sufficient to have a clear view of *either* the context of use *or* the contrast drawn by any specific use to understand the term *in that particular case*. This means that there can be no exceptionless, univocal, accounts of 'dehumanise', 'human-ness' or their cognates. The issue of exceptionless accounts of the meaning of words was addressed through consideration of Baker's (2004) characterisation of Wittgenstein's uses of the term 'metaphysical'. The importance of context can be developed further by looking at the need for occasion-sensitivity and the potential role (and limitations) of ostensive, rather than verbal, definitions in our understanding of terms such as 'dehumanise'. Consideration of such matters will also supplement the discussion above of exceptionless accounts of the meaning of words.

Occasion-sensitivity and Ostensive Definition

In relation to occasion-sensitivity there are two important points to make here. First, I will address the issue of two (seemingly) equivalent expressions which appear to be interchangeable, as a means of illustrating the importance of occasion-sensitivity in our use of expressions containing 'dehumanise', 'human' or their cognates. I will then consider the need for occasion-sensitivity even in cases of the use of a single expression; cases where the same words are used, but not necessarily with the same meaning.

There are many expressions that we are happy to regard as equivalent under *certain* conditions, but would rightly wish to distinguish from each other under different conditions. For example, in many cases we would only cite style as a reason for preferring to say 'There is a pig in the sty' rather than 'The sty contains some ambulatory pork' (Travis 2005, 61).[19] However, when faced with a quadraplegic pig (see ibid.) we see that the two expressions cannot *always* be taken as equivalent. Notice that in many cases it will cause us no problems whatsoever if we treat the two expressions as equivalent, but in some (other) cases we will have to distinguish between the two expressions to avoid misunderstanding. The two expressions describe two different ways that the world can be. This means that while under certain conditions either expression will adequately describe the way the world is *for our purposes*, under different conditions one of the expressions could simply be false and the other true. In such cases, the way the world is provides us with a motive to draw a distinction between the two expressions and determines what would constitute appropriate use of those expressions.

So, in cases of the use of 'dehumanise', 'human-ness' etc. we must always be alert to the impact that the context has on the nature of the contrasts that it is necessary to draw in any given case. In cases where it seems possible to give an exceptionless account of the meaning of 'human' or 'dehumanise', we must be careful that we do not slide into a metaphysical use of those terms.

Yet it is not simply the fact that there are two expressions involved here that creates the need for occasion-sensitivity. This can be clarified by considering another example from Travis (1989, 18 – 19):

> Hugo sits reading the paper. At his elbow is a cup of black coffee. Across the room is a refrigerator, empty except for a puddle of milk at the bottom. Hugo's partner, Pia, says, 'There is milk in the fridge.' To see that this utterance is occasion-sensitive, consider two cases. First, immediately before the moment described above, Hugo, whose fondness for white coffee is legendary – had looked sadly at the coffee cup. Seeing his look, Pia makes her statement: in doing so, she says (falsely) that the fridge contains milk which might be used to whiten Hugo's coffee. In the second case, Pia had previously asked Hugo to clean the fridge – now she finds him reading the paper, drinking coffee and *still* the fridge isn't clean! So Pia utters the sentence, saying (truly) that the fridge contains the puddle of milk.

In the first instance what Pia says is false and in the second it is true. However, nothing in *what she says* has changed. 'Milk' still means milk, 'in' still means inside the fridge.

The indexicals ('here', 'now' etc.) aren't responsible for the change in the truth of Pia's statement either. She is still referring to the same fridge, not a different fridge and/or a different time. In this example, 'milk' makes 'any of an indefinite variety of distinct contributions to what is said in speaking it, and, specifically, to the truth condition for that' (Travis 1991, 242).

In instances of the use of 'dehumanise' there is no finite totality of cases which could be covered by a single (or even two or three) account(s) of the meaning of the term. There can always be problematic cases because what constitutes dehumanisation in any particular case is not an action, form of behaviour etc., but an action in a specific context. As there is no finite totality of possible contexts, then it is not possible to disambiguate through the formulation of a rule for the use of the term 'dehumanise' (say, for example, a rule which said 'we use the term this way most of the time, but in cases such as . . . we use it this way . . ., and in cases such as . . . we use it this way . . .' etc.) (cf. McFee 2004, 47 – 9). There is no way that such an account could be complete in the sense of dealing with *all possible* cases and yet it is perfectly complete *if* it deals with the cases at hand at any given time. The idea of completeness doesn't seem to belong here because it is not only unhelpful but misleading in its implication that there is such a thing as a finite totality of cases which constitute all possible uses of 'dehumanise' and which could be covered by an account of the meaning of the term (see McFee 2004, 52 for a similar discussion in relation to rules).

This is not a matter of the meaning of words, but rather of the way the world is. It is this that makes it necessary to look at the specific details of the case at hand, and makes it impossible to give an account of the meaning of a word that is not in reality an account of the meaning of that word when it is used in specific cases. A consequence of this is the fact that clarification of the context of the use of a term or expression can render the meaning of that term or expression perfectly clear when it was otherwise *seemingly* ambiguous. The reason that it is only *seemingly* ambiguous is that although *the word(s)* can have many different meanings, or at least, contribute to the sense of the expression in any number of different ways, it does not have more than one meaning in *this* specific case. If the meaning is unclear because the context is unclear (say, for example, we do not know who the speaker is in this case) and the meaning becomes clear when we do know who the speaker is, then there was never more than one meaning *in this case*. The problem was that we were not clear on what this particular case was. See Travis (1984, 78 – 81), McFee (1992, 121) and McFee (2004, 50) for a discussion of the difference it makes to know that the instruction 'Bring me a red fish' was given by a marine biologist and not a cook.

An obvious response here is to argue that the problem lies in imprecision of use. One might claim that if Pia's utterance had been more carefully constructed, then it would have been perfectly clear what she meant. McFee (2004, 50 – 1) provides five reasons why this is a poor argument:

1. As noted above, there is not ambiguity *in this case*. All we need is to know what this case actually is.
2. It is not clear how cases might be distinguished. This point can be lost when examples are given in which two ways of understanding an utterance are indicated. This is necessary for clarity, but in reality there are likely to be many more than two possible ways to take an utterance and the number of ways will vary between cases.
3. It isn't possible to say which option is the correct one *on the basis of what is said* even if there are only two possible options. The truth-value of both options is the same. If Pia

says that there is milk in the fridge, that is true if there is a puddle of milk which could not be used to whiten Hugo's coffee, and it is also true if there is milk in the fridge which could be used to whiten Hugo's coffee. The meaning of the words that are spoken by Pia does not make one or other of the options clearly the correct one.
4.   If a term is ambiguous, it must be possible to say in what ways it is ambiguous and also, therefore, in how many ways it is ambiguous. Yet, this does not seem to be possible. There is no finite totality of ambiguities.
5.   Any new, more precise, utterance would still be subject to occasion-sensitivity and this would still not be a consequence of words not meaning what they appeared to mean ('milk' would still mean 'milk' etc.). It is not possible to predict the use of expressions or the correct understanding of an expression, yet we will recognise the correct understanding when we encounter an expression *in context*. McFee (2004, 51 – 2) points out that 'there is no *basic* level of description or explanation' to which we can disambiguate (either up or down). There will always be a sense of a given term which escapes disambiguation and the notion of a finite totality of aspects to the description of any occasion doesn't seem to make sense.

In summary, our understanding of terms such as 'dehumanise' and 'human' is occasion-sensitive because the correct understanding of an expression depends on the way the world is in the particular case at hand, not on the meaning of the words in the expression. Also, different ways in which the world is can render one expression untrue while making another, seemingly equivalent, expression true. Disambiguation is not possible because there is no finite totality of possible misunderstandings of a term or expression. This has two consequences: it raises the possibility that the correct understanding of the term 'dehumanise' on certain occasions may not have the same connection to the term 'human-ness' that it has on other occasions (those highlighted by Schneider and Butcher's (2000, 196) criticism of what they refer to as 'the dehumanisation argument'). Also, it rules out the simple knock-down argument advanced by Schneider and Butcher (2000), because all that is required here is to find one case which does not conform to the general criticism levelled by Schneider and Butcher (2000).[20]

The first of these two consequences can be taken further. Not only does the occasion-sensitive nature of the use of terms such as 'dehumanise', 'human' and their cognates illustrate the fact that certain apparently universal connections between terms do not always hold (such as that between 'dehumanise' and 'human-ness'), but also the function of the prefix 'de-' is not always the same in different uses of the term 'dehumanise'.

When we say that something is dehumanising we often mean that it is degrading. This is far from the same thing as saying that it makes us no longer (or less) human. Notice that the prefix 'de-' in 'degrading' does not tend to produce the same response as it does in 'dehumanising'. In other words, we do not ask what it is that is *lost* when we are degraded as readily as we ask what it would mean to be less or not human.

Consider the following:

'The genetic modification of athletes is dehumanising.'
'By the time they found the body it was badly decomposed.'
'The hurricane caused great destruction.'
'The hostage was decapitated.'
'The troops were demobilised.'

It seems here that 'decompose', 'destruction', 'decapitated' and 'demobilised' are used in a very different way from 'dehumanising'. In all the cases other than 'dehumanising' the 'de-' does roughly indicate a lack of something that previously was the case. This, however, is not *always* the case in relation to 'dehumanising' Someone might say that 'de-' indicates a change of state (in 'decapitated', 'destruction' etc.), but the base morpheme of each term indicates that this is not the case.

The points made here about occasion-sensitivity and the various uses of terms such as 'dehumanise' and 'human' raise an apparent problem – how can one explain the meaning of a word such as 'dehumanise' if a univocal account is inadequate? Put another way – how might we define the term 'dehumanise'? The short answer is that we generally know what is meant by the word 'dehumanise' from the context in which it is used in a given case. There is no need for us to have a definitional account either of what it is to be human, or of what 'dehumanisation' means. A definition in either case appears 'neither possible nor desirable' (McFee 2004, 22). However, the short answer will not suffice. It may be true that we *generally* know the correct way to take terms or expressions from the context of their use, but it is in cases where we *don't* know the correct way to understand a term or expression that we tend to look for a definition. The question remains, what do we do in those cases?

Wittgenstein highlights an important distinction in relation to definitions. He notes that

> What one generally calls *'explanations of the meaning of a word'* can, *very roughly*, be divided in to verbal and ostensive definitions. It will be seen later in what sense this division is only rough and provisional (and that it is, is an important point). The verbal definition, as it takes us from one verbal expression to another, in a sense gets us no further. In the ostensive definition however we seem to make a much more real step towards learning the meaning.[21] (*BB*, 1)

Ostensive definition consists of three features: 'a deictic gesture, something pointed at and a verbal formula (especially "That is ..." or "That is called '...'")' (Baker and Hacker 1992b, 87). For example, McFee (2004, 171) directs us to Wisdom's (1965) example of two methods of explaining what a greyhound is to a child. 'The father's method' involves explaining that a greyhound is 'a dog of such-and-such a type' McFee (2004, 171). 'The mother's method' is to give an ostensive, rather than a verbal definition:[22] 'That's a greyhound, and you remember your uncle's dog, Entry Badge, well that was a greyhound. But now that [she says, pointing to a Borzoi] is not a greyhound, and even that [she says, pointing to a whippet] is not' (Wisdom 1965, 69).[23] This is relatively straightforward when dealing with entities such as greyhounds, but how can ostensive definition work in relation to 'dehumanise' or 'human'? Baker and Hacker (1992b, 87–8) raise three questions which are of relevance if we wish to move from simple cases (greyhounds) to more complex ones ('dehumanise', 'human' etc.): 'what counts as a deictic gesture, i.e. as pointing?' 'What counts as something pointed at?' and 'What counts as an admissible form of words in an ostensive definition?' Pointing to a greyhound, an inanimate object, or even a person is one thing, but how does one point to human-ness or dehumanisation? There are two parts to this problem: is it necessary to actually point? and what exactly would one point to in such cases? As already noted, in the case of human-ness there is nothing to point to, in the sense that 'human-ness' does not refer to a 'thing'. Drawing attention would seem to be sufficient for a deictic gesture and that need not actually entail pointing. The problem of what to point to is reduced when we recognise that a referential approach to language, which takes words as necessarily referring to things or objects, is a central target of criticism for Wittgenstein. It would be necessary to draw attention to some form of behaviour or a state of affairs, not to an essential feature of a person or group of people. Drawing attention to a form of behaviour or state of affairs as dehumanising or an example of human-ness would seem to have the potential to illustrate the meaning one is giving to the relevant term in this particular case at least as well and perhaps, given the points above about occasion-sensitivity, even better than verbal definitions, but there is clearly another problem here. As Wittgenstein warns 'an ostensive definition can be variously interpreted in *every* case' (*PI*, §28). A corollary of this is the fact that an ostensive definition can be variously *misunderstood* in *every* case (Baker and Hacker 1992a, 81). This would seem to be no better than the problems which arise with verbal definitions. However, context is not the only relevant feature that I wish to stress here; there is also the issue of the contrasts that are drawn in specific cases.

A central contention here is that terms such as 'dehumanise' are only used in specific contexts and that this means that there is always a contrast (with human-ness) drawn in any use of the word. Differences in contrasts that are drawn in particular cases lead to a range of ways in which 'dehumanise' is used. Contrasts in use also constitute contrasts in meaning; 'dehumanise' cannot be treated as if it were univocal. Wittgenstein is widely regarded as holding the view that 'meaning is use'. What he *actually* claimed was that 'for a *large* class of cases – though not for all – in which we employ the word "meaning" it can be defined thus: the meaning of a word is its use in the language' (*PI*, §43). 'Dehumanise' is one of those cases in which its meaning is its use, and that means paying close attention to concrete cases and the different contrasts drawn in those cases. It is necessary to address this point to develop a greater understanding of the complexity of concrete uses of 'dehumanise' – in contradistinction to the account implied by Schneider and Butcher (2000, 196) and largely accepted by Miah (2004). While the aim is not to champion the cause of ostensive definition in opposition to verbal definition (the distinction between the two is far too rough for that), appreciation of the function of context *and* contrasts in use will help clarify the need for a significant ostensive element to our understanding of terms such as 'dehumanise' and cure us of the tendency to look for an essentialist, metaphysical account of 'dehumanise', 'human' and their cognates.

Contrasts in Use

The first point which needs to be clarified here is that there are (at least) two distinct uses of the term 'human'. Consider the following:

(1)   'The blood is human.'
(2)   'His lack of feeling was inhuman.'

(1) refers to the fact that the blood is that of a member of *homo sapiens*, and not that of, say, a dog. This seems fairly obvious and the fact that it is obvious is important. We can understand the meaning of 'human' here from the context. As for (2), we do not say that 'his lack of feeling was *not human*.' I suggest that there are two reasons for this – the grammatical reason, we know that it is better to use 'inhuman' rather than 'not human',

and the fact that 'human' here is not being used in the same sense as it is in (1). (1) means that the blood comes from a member of *homo sapiens*, but (2) does not mean that his lack of feeling meant that he was *not* a member of *homo sapiens*. In this context 'inhuman' means something like his lack of feeling showed that he was uncivilised and lacked basic decency, moral standards and emotional empathy. This is a very different use of 'human' than that which is found in propositions such as (1). In the case of (2), it is the *contrast* which tells us what is at stake – to lack basic decency, moral standards and emotional empathy is inhuman, so the opposite is human behaviour.[24]

There are two important points about this rather obvious distinction between human-ness as membership of *homo sapiens* and human-ness as moral agency. First, the use of 'human' to refer to membership of *homo sapiens* should be largely irrelevant in relation to the kinds of cases where actions and situations in sport are described as 'dehumanising'. This would be true were it not for the second point, which is that the apparently obvious distinction between the two uses of 'human' is commonly missed and this is part of the reason why there is such confusion over terms such as 'human' and 'dehumanise'. For example, the metaphysical, essentialist approach to human-ness blurs the distinction between human-ness as behaviour and human-ness as biological. The idea that we need to grasp the essence of human-ness as a first step in moral evaluation is a clear example of confusion over the distinction between the biological and behavioural uses of the term 'human'. It is this kind of confusion that leads to claims such as that made by Schneider and Butcher (2000, 196) about the need to know what human-ness is before we can say what is dehumanising. A similar confusion seems to plague discussions of performance enhancement in sport. When attention moves from the impact of forms of performance enhancement on competitors who face enhanced athletes to the athletes who are enhanced, then often it is unclear whether the supposed moral concern has shifted to one over whether the enhancement has introduced changes to the body of the athlete that are a threat to his or her human essence (whatever that may be). To employ an idea from Wittgenstein (amplified by Gordon Baker), in cases of such confusion those who are confused are operating with a picture which is inappropriate *in that particular case*. This does not mean that such a picture is wrong in *all* cases, simply that it is misleading in the case in which it is causing confusion.

We cannot *not* be human because being human is not a property that we can have or not have in the manner of a bad mood or a strange hair cut. When I say 'Don't treat me like that, I am a human being' the 'am' is not a copula, but an existential verb. For this reason, it would just be misleading to treat 'dehumanising' as meaning to make no longer human; we can't be anything other than human.[25] Confusion of the existential verb for the copula in such propositions reifies human-ness and is the basis of the search for a human essence.[26]

There is a range of different contrasts that appear to be drawn in cases of the use of 'dehumanise'. For example, the following is a rough categorisation of such contrasts. I make no claim for this as an exhaustive list:

- *'Machine'*: Athletes are often taken to be dehumanised because they resemble a machine by either training very hard regardless of the conditions, or because they appear to show no emotion in competition. The contrast with a machine can even be drawn when an athlete performs extremely well with great consistency, although perhaps such cases are more appropriately thought of as drawing attention to the notion of the athlete as an automaton (see below). Moral concerns arise in such cases because the athlete is regarded as not being an agent in the full sense or lacking appropriate emotion (see Hoberman 1992 and 1995; Culbertson 2005).

- *'Technology'*: The perception of the athlete as a laboratory subject often prompts a contrast to be drawn between the human and the technological. The implication is that the athlete becomes a pawn in a scientific game; what is really being tested is not the abilities and qualities of athletes, but technological developments. For example, Hoberman (1992, 195) notes that: 'Over the past forty years Western ideas about the Communist program and its scientific basis have evolved along with Cold War trends. From the beginning, images of the dehumanised Communist athlete have served the psychological needs of populations who doubted the full humanity of all Communists.' This is also the contrast that is drawn in cases where *sports* are regarded as dehumanised by, for example, technological advances in equipment ('Formula One has become dehumanised. All the driver has to do is point the car in the right direction; the thing drives itself').

- *'Unnatural'*: This is closely related to the contrast with technology, but importantly what constitutes the unnatural need not *only* be the use of performance-enhancing drugs, enhancement-surgery or genetic modification. It is equally possible that the heavy training regimes and regimented lifestyles of athletes could be regarded as unnatural (and therefore such practices regarded as dehumanising). This is the contrast with human-ness found in statements such as 'his training regime and whole lifestyle were dehumanising, it's not natural to live like that'.

- *'Automaton'*: This is closely related to the contrast between human-ness and machines. Consistency is a key feature in this contrast. The athlete who consistently performs well is thought of as lacking the failings of humans, which introduce inconsistency into performance. Apparent lack of susceptibility to pain or emotion is another feature of the automaton analogy. The contrast between 'human-ness' and 'automaton' draws attention to a narrower set of features than the contrast with 'machine'. This can be seen in the following example from Hoberman (1992, 55): 'Dehumanizing the black "automaton" while exalting his physical skills, Bache provides yet another example of Western ambivalence toward the biology of the racial alien.'

- *'Cyborg'*: The contrast between 'human-ness' and 'cyborg' is often employed in relation to enhancement surgery, genetic modification and other forms of technological manipulation of the body. Importantly, however, this contrast does not contain all the features of the contrasts between 'human-ness' and 'technology' or 'machine'. It is important to note that the contrast is not usually a literal analogy.

- *'Animal'*: The athlete who appears to lack conventional human capacities to control his or her behaviour, and perhaps also emotions, in competition. Such a contrast can manifest itself in the use of a nickname to refer to the athlete; a name which refers to an animal that displays the characteristics which the contrast between an animal and human-ness highlights.

- *'Monster'*: The contrast here draws attention to *measured* aggression and violence on the part of an athlete, for example, as displayed by self-styled hard men such as former soccer player Vinnie Jones. Such behaviour is much more *deliberate* than that which the contrast between 'human-ness' and 'animal' draws attention to.

- *'Zombie'*: here the contrast draws attention to the emotionless, blank way in which the athlete conducts him or herself. However, this is a narrower contrast than that with 'automaton' or 'machine'.

- *'Mutant'*: The athlete who appears to possess physiological advantages beyond those commonly found even in the most gifted athletes is taken not to be human through a contrast with the notion of a mutant; something is not quite right, the advantage enjoyed by this individual exceeds the normal human range of physiological capacity.
- *'Dupe'*: Applied to the athlete who fails to see that his or her priorities are wrong, and who is duped into doping or other forms of performance-enhancement by overemphasis on the performance principle and/or the logic of quantifiable progress.
- *'Oppressed'*: For example: 'Stalinist dehumanization throughout the Eastern bloc provided a realistic basis for such images [of dehumanised Communist athletes] even as they were embellished by fantasies about the effects of communism on human nature' (Hoberman 1992, 195).
- *'Degraded'*: The athlete whose doping is exposed, or (under certain circumstances) the athlete who is training in a howling gale and pouring rain.
- *'Undignified'*: Again, this is a contrast that can be drawn in cases where doping has been exposed, but also where illness or death is the product of doping and/or other performance-enhancement practices. The collapse and subsequent death of the British cyclist Tom Simpson while climbing Mont Ventoux during the 1967 Tour de France is an appropriate example here. This contrast need not only be drawn in cases of performance-enhancement however. The pitiful state of Paula Radcliffe during both the marathon and the 10,000 metres at the 2004 Olympic Games is another example of where this contrast *might* be drawn.[27]

There is a degree of overlap in this list. For example, a mutant or a cyborg would be regarded as unnatural. Perhaps a monster and a zombie would be regarded as in some way animalistic. An obvious question, therefore, is why distinguish so many contrasts when there is clearly such overlap between them? The significance of the subtlety of these contrasts lies in the fact that the contrasts are drawn in concrete cases and while a contrast between the human and the technological may often seem the same as a contrast between the human and the unnatural, this will not always be the case (cf. Travis 2005, 61). We are on the same terrain as the idea of cluster concepts, or the notion of family resemblance here. Similar contrasts are not identical contrasts, and it is the differences between them that is important. One contrast will draw attention to some, but not all, of the features of another contrast. The specifics of any given case will determine which is the appropriate contrast *in that case*. The important thing in identifying the contrasts with 'human-ness' is the picture, or conception, that underlies that contrast. If we can identify the conception that accompanies the contrast, then we can see how that picture creates an apparent philosophical problem unnecessarily (a strategy similar to that employed by McDowell 1996).

Moral Particularism

The root of the problem here is that an account of 'human-ness' *appears* necessary because there is an implicit prior commitment to general ethical accounts of those features of performance enhancement that leave us perplexed. If a particularist approach is adopted, the *need* for a univocal conception of human-ness disappears.[28] This allows us to approach the concepts of 'human-ness' and 'dehumanisation' in the concrete context of language-in-use without being committed to the view that there are no ethical issues around performance enhancement. We can accept that there are issues, but hold that they are context-specific and can only be treated on a case-by-case basis.

The problem here is not so much the contrast between the human and animals, machines, automata, cyborgs etc. (although some contrasts tend to work better than others, or do so more frequently than others). The problem lies in the fact that these contrasts are drawn in a general way. Any particular contrast is designed to highlight (or reveal) what it is to be human (the human essence, or the essence of humanness – the former being a claim about the being of humans, and the latter being a claim about the meaning of a concept). In the concrete reality of language-in-use contrasts are drawn, but they are not always the same contrast because the sense in which we use the concept varies depending on the concrete case. The question which comes to mind here is Wittgenstein's (*PI*, §293) – 'And how can I generalize the *one* case so irresponsibly?'

Conclusion

By way of conclusion I will directly address the six questions raised at the beginning of the article. First, could there be such a thing as 'an agreed-upon conception of what it is to be human'? The argument presented here is that the concrete use of the term 'human' is context-specific and as a result evades the kind of definiteness necessary for a general agreement on the use of 'human' and, therefore, on what it is to be human. Second, is there *necessarily* a connection between 'dehumanise' and 'human-ness'? Again, consideration of the *use* of 'human', 'dehumanise' and their cognates suggests that such a connection is in no way *necessary*. Third, does the prefix 'de-' *necessarily* function in the same way in 'dehumanise' as it does in 'decapitate'? Once more the response must be negative; it is simply not the case that the prefix 'de-' *always* functions the same way in 'dehumanise' as it does in words such as 'decapitate'. The fourth question, 'Could a human being ever not be, or be less, human?' was, to a large extent, answered immediately after it was posed. In the sense of being a member of *homo sapiens* one cannot be other than human, but in other senses of the term 'human' it is quite possible to suggest that one is not human, or, perhaps more accurately, not *fully* human. That, however, is a trivial point; what is important is the range of different ways that someone might be taken to, *in some way*, not be (fully) human. This is important because it is failure to appreciate the range of ways that we use the term 'human' that leads to the confusion behind claims such as those made by Miah (2004), and generally accepted within the philosophy of sport literature, about the relationship between human-ness and the moral evaluation of performance-enhancement. Fifth, are 'dehumanise' and 'human-ness' *each* univocal? Consideration of the concrete use of such terms has shown that they are not univocal, but can be used in a range of different ways which constitute a range of different meanings. The final question asked if 'human-ness' referred to a 'thing'. In other words, can 'human' be taken as a referential term? In addition, can 'dehumanise' be taken as indicating a lack of that which 'human' refers to? The answer in both cases is 'No'. So the quest for a human essence is futile and misguided and the idea that there is anything about the terms 'human', 'dehumanise' and their cognates that is hidden and requires elucidation by analysis is also incorrect. As Wittgenstein (*PI*, §126) urges: 'Philosophy simply puts everything before us, and neither explains nor deduces anything. – Since everything lies open to view there is nothing to explain.'

So my contention is that the philosophy of sport should abandon the notion that moral evaluation of performance-enhancement is dependent on (i.e. can be validated by) an adequate conception of human-ness. Quite simply, consideration of our use of relevant terms shows the notion of an adequate conception of human-ness to be a fiction, which serves no positive function in the moral evaluation of performance-enhancement. In fact, it serves the wholly negative function of leading us in completely the wrong direction. No satisfactory moral evaluation of performance-enhancement is possible while we are in the grip of the picture which tells us that such evaluation should be founded on an understanding of the nature of human-ness. In addition, we find related confusions, such as Schneider and Butcher's view of the dehumanisation argument, further misleading us in our attempts to gain a clear view of the real nature of the task facing us in the moral evaluation of performance-enhancement.

ACKNOWLEDGEMENTS
Versions of this paper were presented to the British Philosophy of Sport Association Annual Conference, Stanley, Co. Durham, May 2005; the Philosophy, Ethics and Sport Conference, University of New Brunswick, Fredericton, Canada, June 2005; and the International Association for the Philosophy of Sport Annual Conference, Olomouc, Czech Republic. I am grateful to those who commented on the paper on those occasions, particularly Jim Parry, Bill Morgan and Angela Schneider. I am most grateful, however, to Graham McFee, who commented on the paper at length in writing. The paper is significantly improved as a result of his comments. I am responsible for existing weaknesses. I would also like to thank the anonymous reviewers and Mike McNamee for their generosity during the review process.

NOTES

1. Someone might raise the issue of a Parfitian analysis of personal identity here. The instantiation (see Parfit 1984, part three) of my mental processes in non-human corporeal matter could be regarded as making me no longer human, but not preventing me from being psychologically continuous with my previous (human) instantiation. The concern here is that on this view I could be other than human. I am grateful to a reviewer for raising this point. However, it should be pointed out that the position defended in this article would dispute the claim that I can be equated with my mental states and the possibility of the instantiation described above. A detailed discussion of the grammar of 'I' is required to deal with this matter, but it is beyond the scope of this article to provide such a discussion.
2. I am grateful to Graham McFee for introducing me to the notion of a 'trouser-word'.
3. The expression 'wears the trousers' has patriarchal connotations. While I will not completely avoid its use, because it appears in a number of the texts discussed here, I will often replace the expression with reference to the 'dominant' form of a term.
4. I have employed the procedure of using standard abbreviations for the works of Wittgenstein. Many of the quotations from Baker (2004) use these abbreviations.
5. Austin's fourth point (irrelevant for our purposes here) is that 'real' is an '*adjuster-word*' (Austin 1962, 73). In other words, it helps us to deal with indeterminate cases.
6. There are other words that are substantive-hungry. Austin gives the examples of 'the same' and 'one' (Austin 1962, 69). He notes that 'the same *team* may not be the same

collection of players; a body of troops may be one *company* and also three *platoons'* (Austin 1962, 69). There is also the case of 'good'. Austin points out that we must ask 'A good *what*?', 'Good *at* what?' (Austin 1962, 69).

7.   The notion of a 'trouser-word' has been employed by McFee (2004, 135) in relation to 'fair play'. Cf. Baker and Hacker (1980, 79 – 81) on 'complete'. I am grateful to Andrew Edgar for pointing out to me that 'dignity' is also a trouser word.

8.   Cf. Wittgenstein on 'games' and 'number' (*PI*, §§66 – 7).

9.   A central contention here will be that there is no ambiguity because we can understand uses of 'human' and 'dehumanise' either by consideration of the contexts, or of the contrast that is drawn in any specific use of the terms.

10.   Austin (1962, 71) gives the examples of 'proper', 'genuine', 'live', 'true', 'authentic' and 'natural' on the affirmative side, and 'artificial', 'fake', 'false', 'bogus', 'makeshift', 'dummy', 'synthetic' and 'toy' on the negative side. He also claims that 'such nouns as 'dream', 'illusion', 'mirage', 'hallucination' belong here as well.'

11.   The issues raised by Wittgenstein here are very similar to those raised by Heidegger in his critique of Western philosophy. Heidegger claims (1996, §§89 – 101 and 1988, §§10 – 15) that Western philosophy has, since Parmenides (see Heidegger 1992, 130), been dogged by an ontology which is based on the notion of substance (often referred to by Heidegger scholars as 'metaphysics of presence' or 'substance ontology' – see Guignon 1993 and Frede 1993) and as a consequence generates dualisms such as Descartes' *res cogitans* and *res extensa* and Kant's 'noumena' and 'phenomena'. It should be noted that this is *Heidegger*'s position. See Baker and Morris (1996) for an alternative interpretation of Descartes.

12.   See Morris 2004, 1.

13.   Baker points out that not all statements containing 'must' and 'cannot' are taken to be metaphysical (see *BB*, 49) and this is not the only way that statements of essence can be framed (see *BB*, 55 and 66; *PI*, §1).

14.   Baker cites as an example here Wittgenstein's claim that 'when in a **metaphysical** sense I say "I *must* always know when I have pain", this simply makes the word "know" redundant; and instead of "I know that I have pain", I can simply say "I have pain"' (*BB*, 55). The bold text is Baker's emphasis.

15.   Wittgenstein returns to the theme of the lure of scientific accounts for philosophers on a number of occasions. For example, he claims: 'Philosophers . . . are irresistibly tempted to ask and answer questions in the way science does. This tendency is the real source of metaphysics.' (*BB*, 18).

16.   Baker used italics in a quotation to indicate the author's emphasis and bold to indicate his own added emphasis. I have reproduced this in quotations from Baker.

17.   It is not clear whether Miah is considering the word 'human' or some 'thing' called 'human-ness'. If it is the former, then quotation marks would make this clear and if it is the latter, his grammar seems odd.

18.   Fukuyama 2002.

19.   I am grateful to Graham McFee for bringing this example to my attention.

20.   I am grateful to Jim Parry for pointing out the Popperian nature of the task here.

21.   Baker and Hacker (1992a, 37) note that there are many different forms that a definition can take. They argue that 'The classical requirement that definition be a kind of analysis, that it give necessary and sufficient conditions for the application of an expression, was

the product of philosophers' pipe-dreams. It is an illusory ideal that stands in the way of a correct grasp of our form of representation. ... Definitions of a term that analyse it into a conjunction of characteristic marks (*Merkmal*-definition) are only one kind of definition in terms of necessary and sufficient conditions (definitions *per genus et differentiam* are merely a limiting case of *merkmal*-definitions).' They also point out that: 'Definition by necessary and sufficient conditions is only one kind of explanation of meaning, and by no means privileged. It is important to note that contrary to philosophical dogma, different explanations of one and the same term may be equally legitimate. One can define an elephant by genus and differentia, but an ostensive definition at the zoo is not less correct (nor is pointing to a mere picture of an elephant!).'

22.   It is important to remember Wittgenstein's warning that the distinction between verbal and ostensive definition is a rough one. Baker and Hacker (1992b, 87) reinforce this point: 'The class of ostensive definitions has no 'natural frontiers'; it merges imperceptibly into explanations of different forms that might, for certain purposes, be treated as distinct. It is important in philosophy to note that no gulf separates ostensive definitions from *Merkmal*-definitions; there is a continuous spectrum of connecting links. Provided this point is acknowledged, where the boundary of ostensive definition is drawn matters relatively little.' Baker and Hacker (1992b, 89) also point out that ostensive definitions 'shade off into things which are not explanations at all'.

23.   McFee (2004, 172) argues that 'Attempts to force knowledge into the straightjacket of a set of criteria – the sort of thing "the father's method" offered – seem doomed to failure. But this is no cause for complaint, since the mother's method is the typical route to genuine, public, discussible claims – that is, to objectivity. ... And the route is clearly that of particularism ... in line with the commitment to occasion-sensitivity.'

24.   I am grateful to Graham McFee for helping me to clarify my thoughts on this issue.

25.   Wittgenstein was keen to get us to avoid such mistakes. See *PO*, 3; *PI*, 16n, §20, §558, §561 and 149.

26.   This treats existence as a predicate in the sense that it treats human-ness as something which we can lack. The reason that treating *human-ness* in this way constitutes treating *existence* in this way is that we cannot exist as anything other than human. This might seem like sleight of hand on my part – switching from human-ness as dignity, personhood, agency etc. to human-ness as *homo sapiens* in order to reach my conclusion. However, if we reject the notion of a human essence, then we are able to claim that to treat human-ness as something we can lack, under the illusion that there is a human essence, is to treat human-ness (in its real, nonessential form) as something that we can lack. Therefore, to claim that we cannot exist as anything other than human, and to claim that to treat human-ness as something we can lack is to treat existence as something we can lack is a perfectly valid argument.

27.   Of course, many see such cases as examples of heroism and argue that it is the display of such virtues that makes sport valuable. This may or may not be so, but it is irrelevant here. I am not claiming that these are examples of undignified athletes, merely that these are examples of cases where someone might wish to draw a contrast between human-ness and dignity. In that sense, the examples are purely to help the reader see my point. If the examples were to distract in the way outlined above, they would fail to serve their purpose. With that in mind, I offer these examples with reservations.

28.   Someone might argue here that particularism is simply disguised vagueness. This, however, is to misunderstand the point being made here. Something can only lack clarity, or be vague, if it could possibly be clearer. The point here is that any further clarity is impossible and the idea that there is such a thing as a clearer conception which does not introduce the inaccuracies of univocal accounts is a fiction. Pouring two pints into a pint glass does not make the glass fuller; when it contains a pint it is full. The same is true of the terms discussed here; they are not made clearer by identifying a single conception, but rather by identifying the fullest range of possible conceptions because this allows us to consider how the context and the contrast being drawn clarify the term in any particular case.

REFERENCES

AUSTIN, JOHN. L. 1962. *Sense and Sensibilia*. Oxford: Oxford University Press.

BAKER, GORDON. P. 2004. Wittgenstein on metaphysical/everyday use. In Gordon P. Baker, ed., *Wittgenstein's Method: Neglected Aspects*. Oxford: Blackwell: 92–107.

BAKER, GORDON. P. and PETER. M.S. HACKER. 1980. *Wittgenstein: Understanding and Meaning – An Analytical Commentary on the Philosophical Investigations*. Oxford: Blackwell.

———. 1984. *Language, Sense and Nonsense*. Oxford: Blackwell.

———. 1992a. *An Analytical Commentary on Wittgenstein's Philosophical Investigations*. Oxford: Blackwell.

———. 1992b. *Wittgenstein: Meaning and Understanding – Essays on the Philosophical Investigations*. Oxford: Blackwell.

BAKER, GORDON. P. and KATHERINE J. MORRIS. 1996. *Descartes' Dualism*. London: Routledge.

CULBERTSON, LEON. 2005. The paradox of bad faith and elite competitive sport. *Journal of the Philosophy of Sport* XXXII: 65–86.

FREDE, DOROTHEA. 1993. The question of being: Heidegger's project. In *The Cambridge Companion to Heidegger*, edited by Charles B. Guignon. Cambridge: Cambridge University Press: 42–69.

FUKUYAMA, FRANCIS. 2002. *Our Posthuman Future: Consequences of the Biotechnology Revolution*. London: Profile Books.

GUIGNON, CHARLES. B. 1993. Introduction. In *The Cambridge Companion to Heidegger*, edited by Charles B. Guignon. Cambridge: Cambridge University Press: 1–41.

HEIDEGGER, MARTIN. 1988. *The Basic Problems of Phenomenology*, trans. A. Hofstadter. Bloomington, IN: Indiana University Press.

———. 1992. *The Metaphysical Foundations of Logic*, trans. M. Heim. Bloomington, IN: Indiana University Press.

———. 1996. *Being and Time*, trans. J. Stambaugh. Albany, NY: State University of New York Press.

HOBERMAN, JOHN. M. 1992. *Mortal Engines: The Science of Performance and the Dehumanization of Sport*. New York: The Free Press.

———. 1995. Sport and the technological image of man. In *Philosophic Inquiry in Sport,* 2nd edn, edited by William J. Morgan and Klaus V. Meier. Champaign, IL: Human Kinetics: 202–8.

LOLAND, SIGMUND. 2000. The logic of progress and the art of moderation in competitive sports. In *Values in Sport: Elitism, Nationalism, Gender Equality and the Scientific Manufacture of Winners*, edited by Torbjörn Tännsjö and Claudio M. Tamburrini. London: Routledge: 39–56.

MCDOWELL, JOHN. 1996. *Mind and World.* Cambridge, MA: Harvard University Press.

MCFEE, GRAHAM. 1992. *Understanding Dance.* London: Routledge.

———. 1993/4. The surface grammar of dreaming. *Proceedings of the Aristotelian Society* XCIV (2): 95 – 115.

———. 2004. *Sport, Rules and Values: Philosophical Investigations into the Nature of Sports.* London: Routledge.

MIAH, ANDY. 2004. *Genetically Modified Athletes: Biomedical Ethics, Gene Doping and Sport.* London: Routledge.

MORRIS, KATHERINE J. 2004. Introduction. In *Wittgenstein's Method: Neglected Aspects*, edited by Gordon P. Baker. Oxford: Blackwell: 1 – 18.

PARFIT, DEREK. 1984. *Reasons and Persons.* Oxford: Clarendon Press.

POLT, RICHARD. 1999. *Heidegger: An Introduction.* London: UCL Press.

SCHNEIDER, ANGELA. J. and ROBERT. B. BUTCHER. 2000. A philosophical overview of the arguments on banning doping in sport. In *Values in Sport: Elitism, Nationalism, Gender Equality and the Scientific Manufacture of Winners*, edited by Torbjörn Tännsjö and Claudio. M. Tamburrini. London: Routledge: 185 – 99.

TRAVIS, CHARLES. 1984. Are belief ascriptions opaque? *Proceedings of the Aristotelian Society* LXXXV: 73 – 100.

———. 1989. *The Uses of Sense: Wittgenstein's Philosophy of Language.* Oxford: Oxford University Press.

———. 1991. Annals of analysis. *Mind* 100: 237 – 64.

———. 2005. The face of perception. In *Hilary Putnam*, edited by Yemima Ben-Menahem. Cambridge: Cambridge University Press: 53 – 82.

WAISMANN, FRIEDRICH. 1965. *The Principles of Linguistic Philosophy.* London: Macmillan.

WISDOM, JOHN. 1965. *Paradox and Discovery.* Oxford: Blackwell.

WITTGENSTEIN, LUDWIG. 1958. *The Blue and Brown Books: Preliminary Studies for the 'Philosophical Investigations'.* Oxford: Blackwell.

———. 1980. *Remarks on the Philosophy of Psychology*, vol. I. Oxford: Blackwell.

———. 1993. Book review of P. Coffey, *The Science of Logic*. In Ludwig Wittgenstein, *Philosophical Occasions 1912 – 1951.* Indianapolis, IN: Hackett Publishing Company: 1 – 3.

———. 2001. *Philosophical Investigations*, 3rd edn, trans. G.E.M. Anscombe. Oxford: Blackwell.

IS ENHANCEMENT IN SPORT REALLY UNFAIR? ARGUMENTS ON THE CONCEPT OF COMPETITION AND EQUALITY OF OPPORTUNITIES

Christian Lenk

Doping in sport counts as a typical example of unfair behaviour and a good illustration of ethical problems produced by enhancement activities. However, there are some authors who argue that enhancement in sport is not intrinsically problematic but only so in those circumstances that make it dangerous for athletes or unfair to competitors, or which give rise to suspicion in the viewing public. In contrast to this, the author of the present article shows that enhancement activities are contradictory to basic requirements and preconditions of sports competitions. These preconditions are, firstly, a basic equality of opportunities for all competitors and, secondly, a clear causal connection between a specific performance and an individual athlete, in the sense of authorship of that performance. It cannot be excluded that there could exist future sports competitions without these qualities, but this would clearly be a fundamentally different kind of sport from nowadays. Therefore, the normative background of the current concept of sports competitions, as such, limits the use of enhancement practices to a rather low level.

Resumen

El dopaje en el deporte cuenta como un ejemplo típico de una conducta injusta e ilustra bien los problemas éticos que resultan de las actividades de amejoramiento físico. Sin embargo, hay algunos autores que argumentan que el amejoramiento físico en el deporte no es intrínsecamente problemático, sino que es debido sólamente a circunstancias problemáticas que ponen en peligro a los atletas, son injustas para los competidores, y son vistas con sospecha por el público. Contrastando con esto, el autor del presente artículo demuestra cómo las actividades de amejoramiento físico contradicen los requerimientos y precondiciones básicos de las competiciones deportivas. Estás precondiciones son, primeramente una igualdad básica de oportunidades para todos los competidores, y en segundo lugar la clara conexión causal entre el rendimiento deportivo específico y un atleta en particular, en el sentido de autor de tal rendimiento. No puede excluirse que puede que existan competiciones deportivas en el futuro sin estas características, pero esto sería un tipo de deporte fundamentalmente distinto al actual. Por tanto, el fondo normativo del concepto actual de competiones deportivas, como tal, limita el uso de prácticas de amejoramiento físico a un nivel muy bajo.

Zusammenfassung

Doping im Sport zählt zu den typischen Beispielen für unfaires Verhalten, und es ist eine gute Möglichkeit zur Darstellung ethischer Probleme, die durch leistungssteigernde Maßnahmen entstehen. Einige Autoren behaupten jedoch, dass Doping im Sport an sich nicht problematisch sei, es gäbe aber prekäre Begleiterscheinungen, wie die Gefährdung der Athleten, die Unfairness gegenüber den Kontrahenten und der Verlust an Glaubwürdigkeit bei den Zuschauern. Im Gegensatz hierzu, erläutert der Verfasser dieses Artikels, dass leistungssteigernde Maßnahmen den grundlegenden Anforderungen und Vorbedingungen des sportlichen Wettkampfs widersprechen. Diese Vorbedingungen sind erstens eine grundsätzliche Chancengleichheit für alle Wettstreiter und zweitens eine eindeutige Kausalkette von einer spezifischen Leistung hin zu einem einzelnen Athleten, im Sinne einer Urheberschaft. Es kann nicht ausgeschlossen werden, dass es in der Zukunft einen Sport geben wird, der derartige Werte vernachlässigt, aber dieser Sport wäre zu unserem Sport heutzutage grundlegend verschieden. Daher beschränken die normativen Gegebenheiten des aktuellen Sportverständnisses den Gebrauch von leistungssteigernden Praktiken auf ein eher geringes Maß.

摘要

運動禁藥被視為一種典型的不公平行為，而其主要所產生的道德問題，主要是會增進活動表現。不過，有一些作者認為，此一增進活動表現於運動中並不是內部的實質主要問題點，而是基於有問題的環境會使運動員陷入危險情況、產生對對手的不公平，並造成大眾的懷疑情況。與此觀點相反，本文作者認為：會增進表現之活動與運動比賽的基本需求及先決要件產生矛盾現象。首先，這些先決要件為所有比賽者所需要的一個基本公平機會；其次是，一個清楚的隨機連結特定表現與個人運動員的情況，這個觀點為一種原作者之身份。我們不能排除將來的運動比賽可能不會有這些要件存在，但這將會是與現在的運動完全不同。因此，像現行運動比賽概念的規範背景下，是將增進活動表現的使用限制在相當低的層次下。

Introduction

Doping in sport counts as one of the typical examples in discussions on the ethical aspects of enhancement technologies, i.e. non-therapeutic measures that aim to make persons more beautiful, more competitive or better adapted to their social environment. There are an increasing number of such interventions, which may not be welcomed but which are at least tolerated by society.[1]

Typically, the aim of such interventions is the attempt to gain advantages over others concerning the distribution of jobs, hierarchical positions, social contacts, success and acceptance. The practice of enhancement has some problematic consequences. For example, people from ethnic minorities who decide to get rid of their (Asian, African) ethnic identity by plastic surgery also exert an indirect pressure on other people to display a more European appearance. These procedures show an open discrepancy between the practice of discrimination and our ideal of justice, which, in the formula of John Rawls, is one of equality of opportunities – independent from the social or ethnic background (Rawls 1971).

This scenario obviously has something to do with the normative framework in which sports competitions should take place: firstly, we normally expect that there is indeed a kind of basic equality of opportunities between the participating athletes (this seems to be a *conditio sine qua non* for every form of sports competition). Secondly, we find it unfair when single athletes seek advantages in measurements which do not depend on their own performance and training. Thirdly, it is dangerous for sports competitions altogether when athletes put pressure on colleagues to dope themselves by illegitimate methods and produce a kind of biotechnical doping spiral.

The area of sport therefore seems to be a kind of model for society as a whole (cf. de Wachter 2001) – but with stricter demands for fairness and equality of opportunities than in other segments of society. In this field, there remain some open questions which also exist in the case of enhancement in the genuine medical sector: what is a proper definition for doping in sport, i.e. how can we distinguish genuine sports medicine from doping? And why do we accept the enhancement of the technical equipment of athletes, but not of the athletes themselves? Is this maybe a kind of pharmaceutical puritanism, which we should rid ourselves of? These issues will be discussed in the framework of the enhancement debate in medical ethics.

Enhancement: Definitions

One problem in the discussion on enhancement practices is the question of how to define enhancement. This problem seems to be related to the question of what a healthy or 'normal' mental and bodily state is, because the aim of enhancement-practices is mostly described as a kind of super-normal state of body and/or mind.

Eric Juengst's definition of enhancement (Parens 1998a) is very characteristic for this common view on enhancement. It states: 'The term *enhancement* is usually used in bioethics to characterise interventions designed to improve human form or functioning beyond what is necessary to sustain or restore good health' (Juengst 1998, 29).

And this leads to an even older problem in philosophy of medicine – the question of how one could define the concepts of health and disease. It would be hopeless to try to resolve this old discussion here, but there is at least one plausible possibility to describe the objective aspect of health, and this is the functional definition of health from Christopher Boorse: '*Health* in a member of the reference class is *normal functional ability*, the readiness of each internal part to perform all its normal functions on typical occasions with at least typical efficiency' (Boorse 1977, 562).

Obviously, the two definitions above can be used together, and maybe Eric Juengst had Boorse's definition from his 'Theory of Health' in mind when he defined enhancement. The two definitions can be used as preconditions for further arguments on enhancement and equality of opportunities and for answering the question of what would then be a proper definition for enhancement practices in sports medicine. The following definition seems to be appropriate under several aspects: *Enhancement in sports medicine means medical interventions to improve human form or functioning in the context of sports competitions beyond what is necessary to sustain or restore good health*. An example would be the use of anabolic steroids for the building up of additional muscle mass. It is a medical intervention which aims to improve human form or functioning in the context of sports competitions and is clearly beyond therapeutic interventions to sustain or restore the athlete's health.

A functional definition of health seems to be appropriate in sports medicine, because human functioning is the aim of sports medicine, and excellent functioning of human bodies is the aim of sports competitions. Therapeutic interventions in sports medicine would aim to provide good health for athletes (and compensate bodily signs of exhaustion). Enhancement by sports medicine would try to produce extraordinary functioning by medical interventions.

The Significance of Performance and Competition

If one accepts this definition of enhancement in sports medicine as a mere explicative determination, based on an objective (or at least interpersonal) understanding of health, one can distinguish from this the normative background of sport which connects the individual person of the athlete and his performance in sporting contests: *Human form or functioning in the context of sports competitions* should *be improved by the athlete's own training and performance.*

This sentence can be called the 'traditional normative background' of sport.[2] It seems to have something to do with the idea that the winner of sports competitions should justify his individual merits by training and performance (like the author in literature or science should be the person who is responsible for a special work or article), and not by additional technical means which could influence the outcome of competitions. The athlete her- or himself should be the cause of the performance. Enhancement in sports makes it gradually questionable whether somebody won a competition because of her or his own performance or because of other aids. The situation could be compared with students writing an exam: it is permitted for all students to use pocket calculators and encyclopaedias to produce a kind of basic equality of opportunities, but it is not permitted to use aids that directly answer the test's questions such as cribs or reference books, because this would obviously make the written exam worthless. Although the cheating students do in fact answer the questions of the examination, it is not their own original performance that finds the solution to the posed problems. To find out who is for example the fastest runner, one should proceed similarly and define rules for a basic or prima facie equality of opportunities but exclude aids that blur the causality of an individual's efforts to her/his performance. In this sense, de Wachter speaks of an 'equality … that is not a goal in itself but is instrumental for the measurement of the inequality of performances' (de Wachter 2001, 93). De Wachter interprets this constellation not as a psychological or moral attitude of the participants but as a logical requirement of the project to decide which of the athletes performs best:

> The nondiscrimination clause is not an empirical or a normative statement. It is tautological. It expresses the very idea that we want to measure performances. For such a measurement, we have to eliminate all irrelevant factors. In order to discriminate the elements pertaining to a performance, we have to eliminate all elements that are extrinsic to it. (de Wachter 2001, 92)

And 'extrinsic' in this sense means, that nobody should have a mere technical advantage over his competitors.

Ethics and Sport: Code of Ethics and Anti-Doping Code

Ethical considerations are an integral part of current regulations of sports competitions. What do the normative documents of the international sports organisations say on ethics? The IOC *Code of Ethics* demands that

(3) No practice constituting any form of physical or mental injury to the participants will be tolerated. All doping practices at all levels are strictly prohibited....

(5) The Olympic parties shall guarantee the athletes conditions of safety, well-being and medical care favourable to their physical and mental equilibrium. (IOC 2004)

Item (3) can be interpreted from a medical ethics point of view as a variation of the ethical principle of non-maleficence. The focus on non-maleficence raises the question whether there is necessarily a connection between doping practices and doing harm to athletes. This may be not inevitably be the case, but some historical experiences with doping – for example in the former Communist German Democratic Republic – show that doping in sport often leads to doing harm to the athletes (Franke and Berendonk 1997).

Item (5) is a variation of the principle of beneficence and seems to be oriented at the World Health Organisation's definition of health which underlines the subjective aspect of health. It shows that, from the perspective of the IOC, athletes should not only be healthy in the objective sense of the word (i.e. 'normal functioning'), but also feel healthy in the sense of subjective well-being and physical and mental identity and integrity. This seems to be compatible with, for example, a 'safe' kind of enhancement in sport, but not with a perception of athletes that reduces them to in principle variable means to reach maximum performance in sporting contests.

The World Anti-Doping Agency (WADA)'s anti-doping code formulates:

The purposes of the World Anti-Doping Program and the Code are: To protect the Athletes' fundamental right to participate in doping-free sport and thus promote health, fairness and equality for Athletes worldwide....

Anti-doping programs seek to preserve what is intrinsically valuable about sport. This intrinsic value is often referred to as 'the spirit of sport'....The spirit of sport is the celebration of the human spirit, body and mind. (WADA 2003)

Many ethicists will be too sceptical to grant that the participation in doping-free sport is a genuine 'fundamental right'. But personal integrity and autonomy have the character of fundamental rights, and one could argue that the right to integrity and autonomy could justify the absence of doping in sport, in so far that athletes are influenced directly or indirectly to participate in doping activities, especially when these activities are connected with a risk for their health. However, it is not obvious that the athlete's autonomy is endangered in the case of voluntary doping – this seems rather to be a problem of fairness and equality, which also are mentioned in the anti-doping code.

The topics of fairness and equality arise from our behaviour and our ethical duties towards other persons. Equality does not speak as such against doping, because we could suppose a situation where everybody would have the right and the opportunity to dope and enhance himself, and no inequality of opportunities would arise from this situation. The argument from equality speaks only against those situations where not everybody has the opportunity to enhance his bodily functioning in a similar way and to the same degree.

In the other citation, an 'intrinsic value' of sport is proclaimed. According, for example, to the classical Platonic description of 'intrinsic value' in the second chapter of the *Politeia*, it is reasonable that sports activities may have such a value. One does not necessarily engage in sports activities to achieve other goals (gaining popularity or improving one's appearance, becoming a superstar etc.), because sports activities have a value for their own sake (at least for sporty people). The main point of this argument seems to be that sport is a self-sufficient and unproductive activity which is mostly exercised because of its inherent value (pleasure, enjoyment, relaxation) and not to achieve other external goals. It has no external utility in contrast to most other activities on which we spend our day, and this seems to be the main source of pleasure for the ordinary sportsman or -woman.[3] From an ethical point of view, 'the celebration of the human spirit, body and mind' is perhaps a rather awkward description of such an 'intrinsic value'. A better explanation for the 'spirit of sport' could be that one should partake in sports competitions not only for the sake of winning the game (as a so-called instrumental value) but because of the inherent and direct pleasure of sport.

Equality of Opportunities as a Framework for Sports Competitions

In his *Theory of Justice* John Rawls promoted the normative concept of 'equality of opportunities' (Rawls 1971). It is usually applied to problems of resource allocation. Rawls saw a connection between equality of opportunities and his concept of 'justice as fairness'. And it is exactly because of this connection to fairness that there is an obvious analogy between equality of opportunities in the access to societal resources and in sports competitions. Equality of opportunities is clearly less demanding than the equality in the outcome of allocation decisions. On the other hand, it excludes the sheer inequality of opportunities between different persons and parties. Therefore, equality of opportunities seems to say something very important about the structure of sports competitions: many sports competitions exclude outcome equality, because this would mean that there is more than one winning party. But sports competitions need the notion of fairness as a fundamental normative framework, which can be explained as equality of opportunities. Under ideal conditions (none of the athletes is discriminated against or obstructed, each of them has adequate resources and abilities to prepare her- or himself for the competition), equality of opportunities can be interpreted as a mere formal equality which simply prescribes the same rules for all the participants.

Modern liberal societies accept inequality in the allocation of resources as long as it can be demonstrated, however, that inequality of welfare results from inequality of personal performance. When inequality results from unequal opportunities, it is perceived as a kind of 'discrimination'. Therefore equal access to information, welfare and key resources is one of the normative foundations of such societies. The same argument can be applied to sports competitions: inequality in outcomes is not only tolerated but seems to be one of the central goals of sports competitions. Yet the justification for outcome inequality seems to be the basic equality of opportunities. Therefore, rules of sports competitions normally will prescribe the same equipment for all participants and guarantee the same circumstances for all athletes.

Any party who can draw a strong advantage from an inequality of opportunities will be supposed to act unfairly and (mostly) against the rules. If equality of opportunities does not exist, it may happen in sports competitions that the best party not by training and performance but by technical or pharmaceutical preconditions will be the winner. And this would mean that competitions are *unfair* from a structural point of view. Therefore the notion of equality is just as central in sports competitions: every participating party must have equal rights, and no exceptions can be permitted. The important point is maybe rather that there is an approximate equality for each party in the course of sports competitions than the real content of such rules – for example, one could play soccer with ten, 11 or 12 players in each team, as long as the number of players is the same in both teams. In disciplines that include the application of a high degree of technology, such as for example Formula One, sometimes the case occurs that one team is at a substantial technical advantage over other teams. This situation frequently produces a discussion as to whether there should be a stricter regulation of the technical equipment to re-establish a well-balanced equality of opportunities. The reason is that it is just as unfair as boring always to see the same team or person winning because of mere technical circumstances, while the other teams have no realistic chance.

Buchanan et al. (2000) discuss the question of whether there would be a moral obligation to diminish the genetically determined inequality of opportunities by enhancement practices if we had the ability to do so. Their approach was criticised in a recent article by Peter Wenz with the argument that genetic enhancements have an enormous justice-impairing potential (Wenz 2005). Although one could argue for using non-therapeutic genetic modifications for the sake of justice, it seems to be quite unrealistic to expect such an application of enhancement technologies in societies that even fail to balance large inequalities in the access to basic medical services. Savulescu et al. have tried to apply the argument of enhancement as a remedy for genetic inequalities among athletes to the field of sports competitions (Savulescu et al. 2004, 667f). But, as will be discussed below, permitting enhancement practices alone will not necessarily lead to equality of opportunities – worse, it openly decouples the outcome of sports competitions from the athletes' personal training and performance.

Consequences of Permitting Enhancement Activities

The present state of the regulation of sports competitions supports the athlete who abstains from doping and threatens athletes who try actively to get some advantages over others by pharmaceutical means. Allowing doping in sport would produce a new situation, i.e. where those athletes who do not want to be enhanced would have a disadvantage in sports competitions. The decision to accept enhancement practices in sports competitions would therefore drive all athletes to take part in such activities and would make the former concern about the athlete's autonomy senseless.[4] It would give an incentive to the athletes to accept medical or pharmaceutical doping rather than to abstain from it. Otherwise – in a situation where one group of athletes practices enhancement and the other does not – we would produce a new kind of inequality of opportunities, but now with changed roles: in the current situation, one simply has to exclude the use of illegitimate medical and pharmaceutical practices. With athletes being permitted to enhance themselves, a variety of enhancement practices would occur and sports committees would have to decide which degree of enhancement they will accept and how they could produce a new situation of equality of opportunities. This could well lead to the absurd situation where sports committees themselves had to engage in doping research and enhancement activities to guarantee the same technological level for all teams in sports competitions. It is true that the doping ban curtails the autonomy of the doping-prone athletes to enhance themselves – but this seems to be the most practicable (and harmless) solution to produce the decisive equality of opportunities in the concrete situation of a competition.

Competition in Sport or in Technology?

Enhancement practices transfer the competition into the research laboratories. While at the moment we have competition in terms of training and performance, we would likely in the future have a competition in terms of technology, thus dumping safety standards. In a way, this would be very characteristic of our culture, which is technique-prone and accepts a lot of individual risks for the sake of perfect functioning. But it also may produce new risks for the athletes, who will get into a new kind of competition to accept more and more invasive enhancements to their bodies. As argued before, this cannot simply be put aside by the argument for equality of opportunities. Maybe it would be possible to realise equality of opportunities even in an environment that allows far-reaching enhancement practices. In my view, this would produce another consequence, namely, that it would be more difficult (or in some cases unjustified) to identify the athlete her- or himself as the cause of her or his success. This depends on the extent in which doping measurements can influence an athlete's performance. If very effective kinds of doping existed that would enable a totally untrained individual to win sport performances against professional athletes, the pharmaceutical intervention, not the individual her- or himself would be the decisive cause of the success. And this would clearly produce a new kind of sports competitions, maybe more oriented on the technical performance of the whole team (including the team physician), as in high-tech sport such as Formula One. It is interesting to see that there are sports competitions, for example horse races, where it is not the human athlete, the jockey, but the horse who is the real champion. This has obviously something to do with our perception as to who makes the decisive contribution to the race. Enhancement and technological competition could produce new ways to practise sport, but it would clearly be a different kind of sports competition from nowadays, and with a very small contribution by the athlete one could come to the conclusion that she or he is something like a robot, and that the decisive part of the success was produced by the engineers in the research laboratories.

Abstention from Enhancement: Excessive Puritanism or *Conditio Sine Qua Non*?

As historic experiences, especially in the former Communist countries, show, doping practices often do harm to athletes. One example for this is the use of male sex hormones to enhance the muscle mass of both male and female athletes in the former German Democratic Republic. The victims of such practices still suffer from the irreversible damages they achieved (Franke and Berendonk 1997, 1273 – 5). Those practices were clearly unethical because most of the athletes, who sometimes were very young, did not know about these practices and the connected risks and simply took the pills they received from their coaches. This must not necessarily mean that all kinds of enhancement practices will do harm to the athletes, and could be caused by such clandestine techniques and the pressure to act secretly. One could even go so far as to say that the resulting inequality of opportunities was not produced by the practice of doping as such but by the lack of transparency that was caused by the international ban on doping. So maybe it could be possible to construct a kind of ethically 'clean' enhancement that would respect the athlete's health and autonomy and equality of opportunities. For example, some authors even demand the legalisation of performance-enhancing drugs in sport for the sake of fairness and safety (Savulescu et al. 2004).

But those arguments seem to be not very strong in the end. Maybe we should not adopt a position of radical puritanism towards enhancement practices, because there always will be a kind of grey zone between genuine doping activities and enhancement practices that are very closely related to therapy or training.[5] But one important point is that there is indeed a real danger of doing harm to athletes by enhancement – either in cases where the athletes themselves are too ambitious to see the limits past which they would damage their bodies (which would be a paternalistic argument) or in cases where they are forced by unscrupulous coaches and sport bureaucrats to accept more and more invasive forms of enhancement (which would be an argument based on the athlete's autonomy). Moreover, it would be much more difficult to realise equality of opportunities when all kinds of enhancement practices are permitted than in the present state of a general absence of legitimate doping procedures. Sports committees would become a kind of authorising agency for enhancement practices.

Conclusions

What conclusions can be drawn from these arguments? Firstly, a prima facie equality of opportunities seems to be constitutive for the idea of sports competitions. The sense of sports competitions is to answer the question: who competes best in the same circumstances? It is unfair, and should be ruled out, when one party in sports competitions has a decisive advantage not because of training and performance but because of enhancement technologies. Secondly, a basic equality of opportunities could be realised on a lower or higher technological level. Previous experiences with doping in sport show that a higher technological level and more invasive interventions produce often serious risks for the athlete's health and personal autonomy. Thirdly, the technological level influences the degree of similarity between different teams (and hence of equality of opportunities) and of the significance of personal training and performance for individual success. It would be necessary to establish an institution to guarantee the same level of performance enhancement for all teams. This seems to be a worse situation compared with the present state of regulation. Fourthly, therefore, the normative background of the current concept of sports competitions as such limits the use of enhancement practices to a rather low level.

NOTES

1. For example in the area of plastic surgery or cognitive functioning. See the debates on pychopharmaceuticals such as Prozac or Ritalin: Kramer 1994; Elliott 1998; Parens 1998a, 1998b; and Lenk 2002.

2. For examples see the citations in de Wachter 2001, 92.
3. Cf. de Wachter 2001, 90: 'Sport is a form of game. In games we waste time, energy, and ingenuity on pointless and childish tasks. Even the most performance-oriented game remains unproductive. It is all show, a display of excellence for the sake of excellence in activities that are completely irrelevant to life. That which is not, or is no longer, important for "real" life is precisely that which is boisterously celebrated: physical power, skill.'
4. Cf. Morgan 2003, 186f.: 'If steroids were used by *all* athletes in the sport, then the motivation for taking steroids would change. It would become something you were expected to do to ensure fair competition. The shift in motives is important here. . . . I am not taking steroids to take advantage of my opponent. Instead, I am compelled to take steroids because the standards of ethical competition and sportsmanship require me to play to the best of my abilities and fully challenge my opponent. . . . If I am motivated to incur added risk of bodily harm *because* of my moral obligations to the ethics of competition, then it is my moral obligation to incur dangerous health risks. Using steroids is not a free choice to me but rather a moral obligation. This is more than counter-intuitive; it's wrong.'
5. Cf. the recent discussion on the use of hypoxic air machines for training purposes: Spriggs 2005; Tännsjö 2005; Tamburrini 2005.

REFERENCES

BOORSE, C. 1977. Health as a theoretical concept. *Philosophy of Science* 44: 542–73.

BUCHANAN, A., D.W. BROCK, N. DANIELS and D. WIKLER. 2000. *From Chance to Choice. Genetics and Justice*. Cambridge: Cambridge University Press.

ELLIOTT, C. 1998. The tyranny of happiness: Ethics and cosmetic of psycho-pharmacology. In *Enhancing Human Traits*, edited by E. Parens. Washington, DC: Georgetown University Press: 177–88.

FRANKE, W.W. and B. BERENDONK. 1997. Hormonal doping and androgenization of athletes: A secret program of the German Democratic Republic Government. *Clinical Chemistry* 43: 1262–79.

IOC. 2004. Code of Ethics. Available at http://multimedia.olympic.org/pdf/en_report_17.pdf, accessed 11 June 2007.

JUENGST, E. 1998. What does enhancement mean? In *Enhancing Human Traits*, edited by E. Parens. Washington, DC: Georgetown University Press: 29–47.

KRAMER, P.D. 1994. *Listening to Prozac*. London: Fourth Estate.

LENK, C. 2002. *Therapie und Enhancement. Ziele und Grenzen der modernen Medizin* ['Therapy and Enhancement: Aims and Limits of Modern Medicine']. Muenster: Lit Verlag.

MORGAN, L. 2003. Enhancing performance in sports: What is morally permissible? In *Sports Ethics. An Anthology*, edited by J. Boxill. Malden, MA: Blackwell: 182–8.

PARENS, E., ed. 1998a. *Enhancing Human Traits*. Washington, DC: Georgetown University Press.

———. 1998b. Is better always good? The enhancement project. *Hastings Center Report* 28: 1–17.

PLATO. 1979–1980. *Republic*, edited by James Adam. Cambridge: Cambridge University Press.

RAWLS, J. 1971. *A Theory of Justice*. Cambridge, MA: Harvard University Press.

SAVULESCU, J., B. FODDY and M. CLAYTON. 2004. Why we should allow performance enhancing drugs in sport. *British Journal of Sports Medicine* 38: 666–70.

SPRIGGS, M. 2005. Hypoxic air machines: Performance enhancement through effective training – or cheating? *Journal of Medical Ethics* 31: 112 – 13.

TAMBURRINI, C. 2005. Commentary – hypoxic air machines. *Journal of Medical Ethics* 31: 114.

TÄNNSJÖ, T. 2005. Commentary – hypoxic air machines. *Journal of Medical Ethics*, 31: 113.

WACHTER, F. DE. 2001. Sport as mirror on modernity. *Journal of Social Philosophy* 32: 90 – 8.

WADA (WORLD ANTI-DOPING AGENCY). 2003. World Anti-Doping Code, available at http://www.wada-ama.org/rtecontent/document/code_v3.pdf, accessed 11 June 2007.

WENZ, P. 2005. Engineering genetic injustice. *Bioethics* 19: 1 – 11.

WHAT'S WRONG WITH GENETIC INEQUALITY? THE IMPACT OF GENETIC TECHNOLOGY ON ELITE SPORTS AND SOCIETY

Claudio M. Tamburrini

Advances in genetic technology will enable us to intervene in human biological development to prevent and cure diseases, to restore individuals' functions and capacities back to a normal level after injury and even to enhance them beyond what has hitherto been considered as normal functioning for our species. Such a power to reshape and modify the human condition raises fundamental questions that touch upon the central core of morality. One of these questions is distributive justice. Will all people have equal access to the beneficial effects of genetic technology in general and medical genetics in particular? Most of the new therapeutic and enhancement techniques will probably be quite expensive. That means that, probably during a long period of time after the new genetic technology enters medical practice, its use will be practically monopolized by the rich, to the detriment of all those who are not in a position to afford genetic treatments. In this paper, I argue that the health care inequality that inevitably will follow from the adoption of genetic technology, while posing a challenge to provide as long as possible for genetic interventions for all, is hardly a reason to reject the new technology. In that case, we would have to reject any new medicine or medical technique that cannot be made available to all people at once. Finally, I also argue that the 'enhanced new world' that would follow the introduction of genetic technology, even with the kind of inequality that might then arise, poses no serious threat either to elite sports or to society and should therefore be welcome.

Resumen

Los adelantos en tecnología genética nos permitirán intervenir en el desarrollo biológico para prevenir y curar enfermedades, reestablecer las funciones y capacidaces de los individuos a niveles normales después de una lesión, e incluso el mejorarlas más allá de lo que hasta hoy día ha sido considerado como un nivel de fucionamiento normal para nuestra especie. Tal facultad para reformar y modificar la condición humana plantea preguntas fundamentales que llevan al meollo de la moralidad.

Una de estas preguntas concierne la justicia distributiva: ¿Tendrá todo el mundo igual acceso a los efectos beneficiosos de la tecnología genética en general y de la medicina genética en particular? La mayoría de las nuevas terapias y técnicas de mejora serán probablemente muy caras. Esto quiere decir que probablemente durante un largo período de tiempo, una vez que la nueva tecnología genética forme parte de la práctica médica, su uso será monopolizado prácticamente por los ricos en detrimento de todos aquellos que no estén en posición de poder permitirse tratamientos genéticos.

En este artículo argumento que la desigualdad del cuidado de la salud que inevitablemente seguirá a la adopción de la tecnología genética, aunque presentando un desafío para proveer por tanto tiempo como sea posible intervenciones genéticas para todos, no es razón para rechazar la nueva tecnología. De ser así tendríamos que rechazar toda nueva medicina o técnica médica que no pudiera estar disponible para todo el mundo a la vez. Finalmente, también argumento que el Nuevo Mundo del Amejoramiento Físico que resultaría a consecuencia de la introducción de la tecnología genética, incluso con el tipo de desigualdad que podría surgir, no presenta una amenaza seria ni para los deportes de élite o para la sociedad, y consecuentemente debería ser bienvenido.

Zusammenfassung

Fortschritte in der Gentechnologie werden uns in die Lage versetzen in die biologische Entwicklung des Menschen einzugreifen, um Krankheiten zu verhindern und zu heilen, um nach Verletzungen die Fähigkeiten eines Individuums wieder auf ein Normalniveau zu bringen und sogar leistungssteigernd einzuwirken; auch über das hinaus was wir momentan als normales Maß unserer Spezies annehmen. Eine derartige Macht zur Umgestaltung und Modifizierung der conditio humana wirft fundamentale Fragen auf, die zentrale Aspekte von Moralität berühren. Eine dieser Fragen ist die nach Verteilungsgerechtigkeit: Werden alle Menschen gleiche Zugangschancen haben, um von den Möglichkeiten der Gentechnologie im Allgemeinen und der medizinischen Gentechnologie im Besonderen profitieren zu können? Die Mehrzahl der therapeutischen und leistungssteigernden Methoden wird wahrscheinlich sehr teuer sein. Das bedeutet, dass die Gentechnik wahrscheinlich für längere Zeit ein Monopol der Reichen sein wird, zum Nachteil all derer, die sich eine gentechnologische Behandlung nicht Leisten können. In diesem Aufsatz behaupte ich, dass man die Ungleichheiten – die die Einführung der Gentechnik mit sich bringt, solange Sie nicht flächendeckend und für jedermann zugänglich ist – nicht als Grundlage dienen kann diese neue Technik abzulehnen. Wäre dies doch der Fall, müsste man alle medizinischen und medizintechnischen Neuerungen ablehnen, die nicht gleichzeitig allen Menschen zu Verfügung stünden. Und meine abschließende Behauptung wäre, dass die Verbesserte Neue Welt, die durch die Gentechnik entstünde – trotz gewisser Ungleichheiten – keine ernsthafte Bedrohung für den Leistungsport und die Gesellschaft insgesamt darstellt, und diese Technik daher zu begrüßen ist.

摘要

基因科技的突破可使我們介入人類生物科技的發展，進而去預防與治療疾病、在受傷後能恢復個體機能與能力至正當水準，且甚至去提昇超越我們人類一般的功能。像這樣可以重塑並修改人類活動條件的能力也產生一些有關道德上的基本問題。

其中一個問題便是有關分配正義 (distributive justice) 的問題：是否所有人皆會有公平的機會來享有一般基因科技及特定醫學基因的效益？大部分的新興治療法及提昇表現能力的技巧將可能相當昂貴。也就是說，大概要等一段長時間，新的基因科技醫療活動才有可能普及一般人，所以在此以前還是會由富有者所掌握。

在本文，我會主張在健康關照的不公平性基礎之下，我們會無可避免的跟隨採用基因科技，但若一直去挑戰所有可能的基因介入行為，這樣的理由會很難拒絕新的科技。就這個角度來看，我們就必須拒絕任何無法給所有人同時享有的新的醫藥或醫療技術。最後，我也主張，提昇表現的新世界將會跟隨基因技術的引進而到來，即使會有不公平的情況出現，也不會對頂尖運動或社會造成威脅，所以也應加以歡迎。

Enhanced New World: The Impact of Genetic Technology on Elite Sports and Society

Gene technology is a promising research area. Recent developments within this particular field of medicine give us reason to expect that, in a not so far ahead future, we will be able to treat seriously sick people and cure them from already declared pathological states or even to prevent disease. In theory, all existing protein levels in the body may be changed by using gene therapy. As a matter of fact, several sick people have already been treated with genetic therapy with positive results and practically no negative side-effects.[1]

In our assessments of medical interventions, a distinction is usually made between *negative* interventions, which are performed with the aim of curing a disease or eliminating a handicap or disability, *positive* interventions aiming at improving the functioning of a human organism within a natural variation and *enhancement proper*, which aims at taking an individual beyond normal functioning of a human organism. To provide antibiotics to a person suffering from pneumonia in order to cure him or her from this disease would be a typically negative intervention. To give human growth hormone to an unusually small child (merely) in order to increase this child's length would be a positive intervention. To provide a man with three-metres-long legs in order to make him unbeatable in long jump competitions would be a typical example of enhancement.

Genetic enhancement, particularly of the third kind described above (that is, enhancement beyond what is perceived or has hitherto been considered as normal for our species) is seen by many critics as a serious threat to our society, mainly because of its association, justified or not, with the eugenic experiments carried on by the Nazis during the Second World War. This rejection is further reinforced by the evident link between genetic technology and sport practices. As the first gene therapy trials are performed with doping-related proteins such as erythropoietin and growth hormone, the potential misuse of this kind of therapy in a new form of doping ('gene doping') makes individuals reluctant to condone the new genetic technologies in sports and in society in general.

At a societal level, many authors have expressed their concern regarding fundamental questions of *distributive justice*: Will all people have equal access to the beneficial effects of genetic technology in general and medical genetics in particular? Most of the new therapeutic and enhancement techniques will probably be quite expensive.

What are the consequences for the social body of a practice of physical enhancement only accessible to the rich? So a first issue to be addressed is: What are the foreseeable effects of using the new genetic technologies in general medicine *for society*? A second question to be posed is instead related to the effects of genetic technology on sports. Some authors fear that the production of super-human (or rather transhuman) athletes might turn sports into an inhuman activity devoid of any meaning for both practitioners and the public. Are these reasons enough to oppose to the development and utilisation of the new genetic techniques?

In my opinion, they are not. In the first section of this article, I will argue that the health-care inequality that inevitably will follow from the adoption of genetic technology, while posing a challenge to make genetic intervention in all its forms accessible to all people, is hardly a reason to reject the new technology. In the second section, I argue that, although the requirement above seems too demanding, inequality in the use of genetic technology might have consequences that go far beyond the usual implications of unequal distribution of health-care assets. Particularly, focusing on germ-cell modification, I will argue that this kind of genetic engineering is especially problematic, as the changes introduced in people's genome will be passed on to future generations. Thus, after decades or perhaps centuries of substantial genetic modifications, a new race might enter the scene on the planet, living side by side with the retarded *homo sapiens* people descending from all those who could not afford genetic modifications in the past.

Finally, the objection above notwithstanding, I will advance my conclusion that this 'enhanced new world', in spite of its essential inequality, poses no serious threat either to sports or to society and is actually preferable to a world in which no one enjoys the benefits of the new genetic technologies.

Genetic Technology for All?

Introducing the necessary or desired genes, into either somatic or germ cells, will be prohibitively expensive for many people. That means that only those who can afford the new genetic technology will be able to benefit from it. This will probably exacerbate current social and economic inequality, adding biological disadvantages to the already existing inequalities between the poor and the rich.

So, an egalitarian might ask, is it not unjust to sacrifice disadvantaged groups in society in order to make new medical advances available for the better-off?

I believe that, as it is formulated in terms of two different social groups with opposed interests, the present objection is misleading. To begin with, the scenario depicted in it, although realistic, is not even new. Historically, the adoption of new medicines and medical techniques has often taken place in a socio-economic situation of inequality. Antibiotics, to name an example, were not available to the poor when they were discovered. But after decades of expansion and development of medical and pharmacological techniques, together with the consolidation of the welfare state, antibiotics are now available to the majority of the world population, regional inequalities notwithstanding. By the same reasoning, genetic technology will no doubt be available to the poor, although not for the *contemporary* poor. Disadvantaged groups will not have access to the new technology at the moment of its introduction, and perhaps this will remain so for decades. But in the future, the use of medical genetics will probably reach the poor strata of society, who will then be able to enjoy the benefits of the new techniques. Thus even if we accepted the terms in which this criticism is cast, the poor would not be 'sacrificed' only to benefit the rich: future poor people get the benefit as well. Seen from this perspective, the present objection loses much of its intuitive appeal. Normally, we do not object to a practice that implies giving less weight, or even ignoring, present people's interests to benefit the worst off in the future.

It should be underlined that, in the particular scenario we are discussing, the alternative that probably would appear as most plausible to egalitarians yields counterintuitive results. To argue that the rich should pay the bill instead of the (present) poor means either that we renounce *developing* the new genetic technology (in which case we would be paying attention to the interests of present poor people, but at the price of renouncing the benefit to future poor and better-off people), or that we *wait to use* the new techniques until we can offer them to all social groups on equal terms (in which case we would be denying a benefit to present better-off people by using an already existing technique, simply to honour a principle of distributive justice which is far from being embraced by all). I find none of these positions defensible.

'Genetic Technology is Different!'

There is, however, a powerful objection to the preliminary conclusion advanced in the previous section. It runs as follows. Genetic technology is different. Particularly when applied to germ-line cells, unequal access to the new technologies might lead to serious social problems of a magnitude never experienced before. As enhanced physical traits will be inherited by genetically modified individuals' offspring, a new class of human beings will develop with physical characteristics clearly superior to those possessed by non-enhanced exemplars of the human species. As a matter of fact, they will be endowed with phenotypes and genotypes not shared with their genetically contemporary 'ancestors' with whom they might even not be able to mate. Thus the unequal implementation of the new genetic technologies might originate a new transhuman species living simultaneously with human exemplars of the old un-enhanced kind (McNamee and Edwards 2006; McNamee 2007).

This is an impressive objection indeed. But how lethal is it really for the new genetics? To answer that question, two different fields of application should be distinguished: (a) elite sports, and (b) society in general. I intend to refer to the latter objection in the next section. In the present one, I will discuss how the prospect of transhumanism might affect elite sports.

Spoiled Sports?

Would the new genetic technologies, followed by the eventual creation of a new transhuman species, spoil elite sports? Is this scenario contrary to the ethos of elite sports? At least at first sight, this is not obviously so. The ethos of elite sports (to be distinguished from recreational sports) might be summed up in the following criteria: (1) to perform at the top of one's capacity; (2) to entertain the public; and (3) to transcend the limits of what hitherto was perceived as possible for humans to perform, physically and mentally. To these conditions, it might be added a fourth one, which is usually meant as a constraint to the pursuit of the goals defined by the three conditions above: (4) sport contests should be characterised by fairness.

Regarding (1), genetically enhanced athletes will perform at levels never dreamt of before, which most probably will increase the sport fans' fascination with the activity (condition (2)). Further, as genetic modifications probably will level out differences in performance capacity established by birth, athletes' initial conditions will be more equal than they are at present. Thus, related to condition (4), sport competitions will probably turn out to be fairer. And, with the physical conditions mainly equalised for all elite athletes, there will be more room for morality in this enhanced new (sport) world. The outcome of the competition will in a larger scale than today be decided either by moral and intellectual excellence (effort, willingness to pursuit a goal and the mental strength and capacity to achieve it etc.) or by unforeseeable casual factors (such as the athlete's condition on competition day or other uncontrollable situations acting on the outcome of the contest). Particularly this latter element might add to 'the sweet tension of uncertainty' (following the expression of Warren Fraleigh), to the delight of the public.

Some critics might argue that this picture of the probable effects of genetic modifications on elite athletes is too optimistic. Once those physically inferior by birth started to catch up with their naturally privileged competitors, the latter will no doubt resort to the new genetics to restore their initial advantage. So the performance gap will increase again, making thereby evident the self-defeating character of widespread and continuous enhancements.

This is indeed a crucial point in my argument. I have already discussed elsewhere a similar objection regarding women athletes' possibilities to catch up with men's sport performance (Tännsjö and Tamburrini 2005). There, a conjecture was made 'that if, in a certain area, one sex is genetically disadvantaged, then, in this area, it is easier for the disadvantaged sex to catch up with the advantaged one than it is for the more advantaged one to move further ahead' (ibid., 188). I believe the same argument might be made regarding transhuman athletes. If this conjecture is tenable, it means that genetic enhancement is indeed a feasible means of levelling out differences.

But how plausible is this conjecture? This question is difficult to answer at the present stage of scientific knowledge. However, there seem to be biological limits to human physical performance. It is probable that will be the case with transhuman physical capacities as well.

Further, there is another consideration counting in defence of the conjecture above. Regarding the gap between female and male athletes' performances, we have argued that

> If gene therapy should be allowed, there are restrictions with respect to security on how it can be used. This means that there must certainly be limitations to what kind of changes could legally be made. A way of setting such limits would be to set limits to muscular mass, haemoglobin concentration in the blood (already implemented in some sports) and so forth. Up to a certain limit it is free for anyone to enhance his or her physical or physiological characteristics. If you go beyond this limit, you are disqualified from the competition. Such a measure would have, as a not intended but clearly foreseeable side-effect, that it would be easier for the sex that is behind to catch up with the other sex than it is for the other sex to move further ahead. (Tännsjö and Tamburrini 2005, 189)

Again, the same argument might be made about transhuman athletes. And once such limitations are enforced, the conjecture gains in credibility. Finally, what kind of sports world will evolve when the new genetics is given free room to develop? Is the transhuman world depicted above compatible with the ethos of elite sports?

In my view, it actually is. An implicit goal of elite sports activities has always been to further the gap between athletes and common people. (In my view, this is the most reasonable interpretation of condition (3) above). The larger the gap, the greater the fascination we feel for those who extend the boundaries of human nature. As a matter of fact, elite athletes already are different from 'normal' people in the sense that they possess physical aptitudes not shared by non-sporting people. The transhuman sporting world would only make that gap more evident. Thus, rather than being incompatible with elite sports, I believe a transhuman world embodies its true spirit.

What's Wrong with the Enhanced New World?

Genetic enhancement, particularly of the third kind described at the beginning of this article (that is, enhancement beyond what is perceived as normal for our species) is considered by many critics as a serious threat to our society. Mainly, their reasons have to do with: (a) the autonomy of self- and other-regarding (for instance, on behalf of our offspring) decisions regarding genetic enhancements; and (b) the supposed reinforcement of suspect cultural values implied in designing a perfect human exemplar, which should remind us of such horrible social experiments as the Third Reich of the Nazis. Thus, the possibility of enhancing human traits through genetic technology confronts us with many troublesome ethical questions that touch upon central notions of morality.

Autonomy

Regarding the objection from autonomy, I believe however that it is not reasonable to conclude from this objection that individuals' decisions will automatically become non-autonomous. Autonomy can be impaired in two different senses (see Tamburrini 2005, particularly 82 – 5). To begin with, it can be argued that individuals are autonomous when they can entertain different courses of actions without impediments. Then a person might be more or less autonomous, depending on the number and degree of activities she or he is able to undertake. Suffering from a serious handicap as a consequence of genetic interventions that went wrong would then diminish the affected person's autonomy. Or so could it be objected to the new genetic technologies.

Now, I have been assuming throughout this article that genetic technology will be implemented once it has been widely tested in medicine and proved to be relatively safe. So, at least in this particular meaning of autonomy, the present objection does not hit the mark.

According to a second notion of autonomy, a person is autonomous to the extent that she or he can decide on her/his life projects, goals, plans etc. It cannot be denied that individuals will be put under a pressure to enhance in the new world of genetic enhancement. But in my view, regarding somatic genetic modifications, this criticism is too wide to qualify as a conclusive objection to genetic enhancement of our physical capacities. In a sense, all kinds of enhancements that go well put a pressure on others to emulate the positive intervention that has been performed on the patient/client. Shall we for instance oppose efficient educational programmes on the grounds that, due to their success, they will push others to go through them and get 'culturally enhanced'?

It is instead regarding genetic intervention at the embryonic level that the present objection seems to be most tenable. Embryos cannot choose for themselves. So, if parents or tutors were to design their physical traits and capacities in advance, wouldn't they be manipulating those future lives in an ethically improper way?

I do not think so. Concerning autonomy, the relevant issue is not whether the improvement was made with the individual's consent or not. Rather, the issue is whether the individual retains her/his capacity to choose freely which path of life to pursue. Provided genetic enhancement adds to the capacities and aptitudes possessed by the individual without neutralising or annulling others, I see no problem in widening the individual capacity repertoire in this way. To provide for the individual's possibility of making her/his own decision on the kind of life (including career choices) she/he wants to live is what distinguishes a good education from bad one. The same criteria can be applied to design an acceptable policy of genetic enhancement.

There is, of course, the question of whether it will ever be possible to simply add aptitudes to individuals, without either risking submitting them to injury or annulling other capacities. That question, however, is for natural scientists and the medical profession to solve. Provided it is satisfactorily solved in the future, I see no objection to genetic enhancement that could be raised from an autonomy point of view.

The Objection from Elitism

What about the charge that genetic enhancements might reinforce suspect, elitist cultural values? In the wake of genetic technology and medical genetics, improvements in both educational skills and physical abilities will inevitably follow. The context, therefore, is already settled by current scientific developments. Perhaps there is something wrong with this development. It might lead, for instance, to the creation of a new, superior species endowed with better tools to cope with the circumstances of life than we have at present. This, however, is not necessarily to the detriment of others. Depending on how it is implemented, such a development might even turn out to be beneficial for other people than the enhanced individuals themselves.[2] It is true that inequality will probably be increased in an enhanced new world. But if, as it was argued in the first section, everyone who can be benefited by it will in fact be benefited, I think the burden of the proof should be put on those who wish to stop the new technologies.

Athletes as Role Models

Finally, it might be argued that genetically enhancing *elite athletes* would be particularly problematic, due to the importance they have as role models for the young. In a world in which athletes become transhumans (or, rather, super-humans), this might be interpreted by the younger generation as a signal that the weak, the ugly or the less intelligent should be despised.

I think we should not exaggerate the impact on the young that a genetically enhanced sport world might have. Rather than cementing fascistoid attitudes among them, I believe we will probably witness the definitive discredit of *commercialised* elite sports. Even more than today, it will then become a freak show. There will always be people who feel attracted by such a spectacle. But that attraction is not massive enough to become a social problem. Quite the contrary: it might even be expected that as a consequence of such a development, people will choose to spend their time practising recreational sports instead of expressing their ethically dubious admiration for the winner in commercialised sport arenas. In my view, it is highly improbable that such a development would be noxious for society.

Conclusions

Humans have always strived to improve their physical condition. In the past this was done by following dietary prescriptions or performing physical training. More recently, the possibility arose of achieving physical improvements by resorting to different drugs and surgery interventions, as the flourishing of the pharmaceutical industry and cosmetic surgery bear witness. In the wake of the new medical technologies, there is now a prospect of attaining the same results, or probably even better, in this eternal quest for improvement by means of genetic enhancement. In this article, I argued that a traditional objection to such a development – namely, that it adds an unequal distribution of genetic assets to already existing socio-economic inequalities – is not strong enough to be taken into account. Usually, we approve of policies that imply putting reasonable burdens upon present generations in order to benefit future people. Particularly, this seems ethically commendable when the poor are among those who will be benefited in the future. This applies, I have argued, to the implementation of the new genetics. No objection is therefore to be addressed to genetic technology on distributive grounds.

And the prospect of a new species coming onto the historical scene should not frighten us either. Look around and see the reality surrounding us. Are we really warranted in fearing things could become worse?

ACKNOWLEDGEMENTS

I wish to thank the participants of the workshop on physical enhancement arranged by the Stockholm Bioethics Centre at Oxford in May 2006 for their helpful comments on an earlier draft of this article.

NOTES

1. At present, more than 3,000 patients have been treated with some form of gene therapy, with very little side effects. The treatment was applied to a number of different diseases ranging from cancer to heart failure. Recent clinical data show encouraging gene therapy results in three major diseases, the first two being patients with x-linked severe combined immunodeficiency disease (Cavazzana-Calvo et al. 2002) and patients with hemophilia B (Manno et al. 2000). Thirdly, angiogenic gene therapy with vectors expressing the human vascular endothelial growth factor for the treatment of coronary artery disease showed improvement in angina complaints (Losordo et al. 2002). The conclusion suggested by these studies is that gene therapy is generally a safe treatment with a potential for curing patients with, in some cases, life-threatening diseases when no other treatment alternatives available. All these data are gathered from H.J. Haisma's report presented at

the Stockholm Bioethics Centre workshop on Physical Enhancement within the European Enhance-project on 5 May 2006 at Oxford (Haisma 2006).

2. What I have in mind here is the prospect of developing individuals, or a new species, with improved empathy and social engagement.

REFERENCES

CAVAZZANA-CALVO, M., S. HACEIN-BEY-ABINA, F. LE DEIST, F. CARLIER, C. BOUNEAUD, C. HUE, J.P. DE VILLARTAY, A.J. THRASHER, N. WULFFRAAT, R. SORENSEN, S. DUPUIS-GIROD, A. FISCHER, E. GRAHAM DAVIES, W. KUIS and L. LEIVA. 2002. Sustained correction of Xlinked severe combined immunodeficiency by ex vivo gene therapy. *The New England Journal of Medicine* 346: 1185 – 93.

HAISMA, H.J. and O. DE HON. 2006. Gene doping. *International Journal of Sports Medicine* 27: 257 – 66.

LOSORDO, D.W., P.R. VALE, R.C. HENDEL, C.E. MILLIKEN, F.D. FORTUIN, N. CUMMINGS, R.A. SCHATZ, T. ASAHARA, J.M. ISNER and R.E. KUNTZ. 2002. Phase 1/2 placebo-controlled, double-blind, dose-escalating trial of myocardial vascular endothelial growth factor 2 gene transfer by catheter delivery in patients with chronic myocardial ischemia. *Circulation* 105: 2012 – 18.

MCNAMEE, M.J. 2007. Whose Prometheus? Transhumanism, technology and the moral topography of sports medicine. *Sport, Ethics and Philosophy* 1 (2): 181 – 94.

MCNAMEE, M.J. and S.D. EDWARDS. 2006. Transhumanism, medical technology, and slippery slopes. *Journal of Medical Ethics* 32 (9): 513 – 8.

MANNO, C.S., M.A. KAY, M.V. RAGNI, P.J. LARSON, L.B. COUTO, A. MCCLELLAND, B. GLADER, A.J. CHEW, S.J. TAI, R.W. HERZOG, V. ARRUDA, F. JOHNSON, C. SCALLAN, E. SKARSGARD, A.W. FLAKE and K.A. HIGH. 2000. Evidence for gene transfer and expression of factor IX in haemophilia B patients treated with an AAV vector. *Nature Genetics* 24: 257 – 61.

TÄNNSJÖ, TORBJÖRN and CLAUDIO TAMBURRINI. 2005. The genetic design of a new Amazon. In *Genetic Technology and Sport – Ethical Questions*, edited by C. Tamburrini and T. Tännsjö. London and New York: Routledge: 181 – 98.

TAMBURRINI, CLAUDIO. 2005. Educational or genetic blueprints, what's the difference? In *Genetic Technology and Sport – Ethical Questions*, edited by C. Tamburrini and T. Tännsjö. London and New York: Routledge: 82 – 90.

WHO'S AFRAID OF STELLA WALSH? ON GENDER, 'GENE CHEATERS', AND THE PROMISES OF CYBORG ATHLETES

Kutte Jönsson

In this article, I argue that there are moral reasons to embrace the construction of self-designing and sex/gender-neutral cyborg athletes. In fact, with the prospect of advanced genetic and cyborg technology, we may face a future where sport (as we know it) occurs in its purest form; that is, where athletes get evaluated by athletic performance only and not by their gender, and where it becomes impossible to discriminate athletes based on their body constitution and gender identity. The gender constructions within sports and sports culture are solid, however. Here, I argue that the rough distinctions we use to define people in terms of sex/gender tend to create and recreate old-fashioned and discriminatory sex/gender-boundaries. A morally reasonable way of meeting this issue, is to say that the problem is not the individuals who (for one reason or another) transcend certain gender categories, but the categories in themselves.

Resumen

En este artículo argumento que hay razones morales para adoptar la construcción de atletas "ciborgs" [seres parte humana parte máquina] que se autodiseñen y que sean de género/sexo neutro. De hecho, con la perspectiva de una tecnología genética y cyborg avanzada puede que encaremos un futuro donde el deporte (tal y como lo conocemos) ocurra en su forma más depurada; esto es, donde los atletas sean evaluados sólamente por su rendimiento deportivo y no por su género, y donde sea imposible discriminar entre los atletas en base a su constitución física y su identidad sexual. Las construcciones de género sexual dentro del deporte y la cultura deportiva son sólidas, sin embargo. Aquí argumento que las crudas distinciones que utilizamos para definir a las personas en cuanto a su sexo/género tienden a crear y recrear límites de sexo/ género viejos y discriminatorios. Una manera moral razonable de encarar este asunto es el decir que el problema no radica en los individuos quienes (por una razón u otra) trascienden ciertas categorías de género, sino en las categorías mismas.

Zusammenfassung

In diesem Artikel behaupte ich, dass es moralische Gründe gibt warum die Herstellung von geschlechts- und genderneutralen Cyborg Athleten begrüßenswert ist. Und zwar werden wir durch die Weiterentwicklung der Gen- und Cyborgtechnologie in Zukunft Sport (so wie wir ihn kennen) in Reinform erleben, d.h. die Athleten werden nur nach ihrer Leistung und nicht nach Geschlecht beurteilt, was im Übrigen auch die Diskriminierung aufgrund körperlicher Merkmale und geschlechtlicher Identität unmöglich macht. Allerdings die geschlechtskonstruierenden Mechanismen im Sport und der Sportkultur sind recht stabil. Hierbei behaupte ich, dass die Grobeinteilung von Personen in Bezug auf Sex/Gender dazu führt jene altbackenen und diskriminierenden Sex und Gender Grenzen zu produzieren bzw. wieder auferstehen zu lassen. Eine moralisch akzeptable Art mit diesem Problem umzugehen besteht in der Feststellung, dass das Problem weniger bei den Individuen zu suchen ist, die (aus welchen Gründen auch immer), gewisse Geschlechterkategorien transzendieren, als vielmehr in den Kategorien selbst.

摘要

在本文，我主張有一些道德理由可以環繞在自我-設計 (self-designing) 與兩性/性別中立的電子裝置運動員 (cyborg athletes) 之建構上。事實上，在基因工程與電子科技的發展前景下，我們可能會會面臨到未來的運動 (就我們知道) 會成為全然的單純型式表現，也就是說，運動員僅由運動表現來評量，而無去考慮到性別差異，這樣就會便成我們無法去辨識運動員的身體組成及性別身份。不過，性別組成在運動項目與運動文化中的區分在目前還是相當堅固的。在此，我主張我們這種現行有關性別/兩性的粗糙區分法會造成或重塑性別/兩性之間較古板的隔閡樊籬。用合理的道德思維來思考此一課題，便是，這個問題不是基於個人(就一個理由或其他理由)來超越特定的性別分類，而是在於分類本身的問題。

Introduction

In 1980, a 69-year-old woman was accidentally killed by robbers in the parking lot of a discount store in Cleveland, USA. Very few would have known about this tragic incident if it had not been for the victim's identity.

The victim was the Polish-American former runner Stella Walsh, one of the most successful athletes in athletics during the 1930s and gold medallist at the women's 100 metres in the 1932 Olympic Games in Los Angeles. The autopsy of her body revealed that she had been hiding a secret. As it turned out, 'she' was a 'he'.

In the aftermath of this quite spectacular story, one might ask if Stella Walsh was cheating her way to athletic success. Those who argue that she was, usually claim that she was competing under 'false flag'. She was not what she claimed to be in terms of sex. But this is a rather simple statement. In fact, this issue goes much deeper than to what the medical expertise claim to be biologically relevant in a sports context. For instance, the 'fact' that Stella Walsh was a 'man' does not say much about whether she should be accused of cheating. To say that someone is cheating implies, at least according to the usual definition of cheating, that the cheater intentionally acts in a way that gives the cheating athlete an unfair advantage on fellow competitors. In the case of Stella Walsh it is not obvious that she gained an *unfair* advantage based on her sex belonging; in fact it is not obvious that she had an advantage at all.

Of course, Stella Walsh was not genetically manipulated or modified. But suppose she had been. Would it make any moral difference? In other words, is there a moral difference between a 'natural born "cheater"' and an 'artificially constructed "cheater"'?

I will here suggest that this distinction is invalid. In fact, to say that athletes such as Stella Walsh were cheating seems unfair. Because it would be to say that the problem was her body constitution and not the social and cultural construction of gender.

Of course, this issue also concerns the construction of gender within a medical discourse. Some would say that a medicalisation of bodies is occurring. Such a medicalisation can be gendered in different ways, also in the sports context. However, it is possible that the main ethical problem does not lie in the medicalisation as such, but rather in the gender constructions.

Based on this, I will argue that the rough distinctions we use to define people in terms of sex/gender tend to create and recreate sex/gender boundaries, and that this is the foundation of sex/gender-based discrimination in sport. In other words, I will argue that the problem of gender discrimination comes with the gender categories in themselves, and not with the individual athletes who may challenge and transcend certain gender boundaries with their bodies and identities. To this, I will suggest that we have moral reasons to embrace the construction of self-designing and sex/gender-neutral *cyborg athletes*.

Three Types of (Disciplinary) Sport Technologies: Performance-enhancing Technologies, Surveillance Technologies and Gender Technologies

'[S]port performance is wholly the result of technological intervention', Debra Shogan says and continues: 'Performance in sport could not be achieved without organized, systematic, expert application of techniques, mechanisms, or practices that are designed to produce change' (Shogan 2002, 94).

I think Shogan is right. And with that in mind, I will here presume that there are three main types of technologies that can be combined in sport: (a) *performance-enhancing technologies*, for example training equipments, training methods, nutritional supplements, medicines and so on; (b) *surveillance technologies*, for example technological equipments in order to guarantee fair competitions, such as goal cameras, advanced time-keepers and doping tests; and (c) *gender technologies*, that is, technologies that can be applied in order to maintain certain power structures between men and women based on men's and women's respective supposed body structures (Larsson 2005).

I suggest that these three types of basically disciplinary technologies interrelate to each other in sports, but in different ways. For instance, we usually accept *performance-enhancing technologies* and *surveillance technologies* because they serve the interest of constantly improving athletic performances, although not unconditionally. Sport society has banned some of the possibilities of athletic improvement, for example by banning what the International Olympic Committee (IOC), for instance, defines as doping. But, as Gunnar Breivik puts it: 'In modern sport the key element in the various definitions of doping has been the notion of artificial improvement of performance. There have been several problems with such a general definition. What is "artificial"?' (Breivik 2005, 168).

Gender technologies can easily be intertwined with the other types of technologies. For example, both performance-enhancing technologies and surveillance technologies can be used to maintain gender discrimination, for example, by not letting women become 'as strong as men', based on reasons we find to legitimate surveillance technologies.

Moreover, when sport society claims that it is unfair for men and women to transcend the well-defined gender categories, it tends to use arguments of fairness to support that claim. In order to keep the competitions fair, sports society has to control the athletes. Now the gender discipline can be discovered in many of the most basic principles in the logic of sports.

Consider, for example, the principle of fair play. Fair play is a moral norm and a virtue in sport (see for example Loland 2002). It would be easy to say that this principle is gender-neutral. Historically, it is not. In fact, the sociologist Richard Giulianotti claims that what he calls 'the myth of fair play' plays a central role in the reproduction of masculinity hierarchies (Giulianotti 2005, 81). But the principle is leaking in various ways.

Sometimes the leakage takes the form of non-legal violence between athletes on the playing field, sometimes in the use of illegal performance-enhancing drugs; and if we, for a second, widen the concept so that it also includes spectators, sometimes it takes the form of hooliganism. But the leakage also – sometimes – takes the form of athletes who transcend the rather specific gender categories.

The leakage does not interfere with existing sport ideals in an obvious way. For example, hooliganism can be seen as a confirmation of organised masculine violence and doping can be seen as a reinforcement of physical enhancement and as a foundation for athletic excellence. In other words, hooliganism as well as doping can be seen as caricatures of already accepted sport norms. The issue of transcending gender categories is more complicated in this sense. In challenging traditional gender norms, the gender norms are being exposed, which can lead to repressive acts against those who transcend them. In other words, technologies used to keep competitions fair and 'morally sound' work perfectly well as gate-keepers so that athletes do not transcend the traditional gender categories and become 'monsters', that is, characters who challenge the male/female dichotomy. The gender equality issue in sport has been debated for a long time.

Most people seem to accept the division between men and women in sport. The arguments in favour of sex/gender-segregation are usually based on principles of equality and fairness. This goes for feminists as well. In fact, most feminists in sports theory seem to accept the division between men and women, usually for strategic reasons. But does the division really serve the principles of equality and fairness in sports?

Equal Opportunities, Fairness and 'Gender Cheating' in Sport

Let me return to the story of Stella Walsh. Some have argued that she had been cheating. In one way this may be true. The rules in most sports do not allow 'men' to compete in women's sports.

If the IOC had known that Walsh was a 'man' they would not have let her compete. I believe many would have supported such a decision, for example the biologists Katarina Nordqvist and Annika Eriksson.

In an article in the Swedish popular science magazine *Forskning & Framsteg*, Nordqvist and Eriksson (2004) argue that Walsh was in fact cheating. Their arguments are straightforwardly biological. They argue that Stella Walsh had more muscle mass than other female competitors, and in terms of body constitution she was 'like a man'. Therefore, she had an *unfair* advantage over her fellow competitors. (Moreover, they claim that in pictures, she looked 'guilty'. In other words, they are implying that she was *intentionally* cheating.)

Is this a strong argument? I think not. I believe it is more reasonable to say that Stella Walsh 'fell between chairs'. More exactly, she fell between the concept of sex and the concept of gender. This point, I would say, is not irrelevant in terms of fairness in sport. Those who think that she was cheating argue that she was *too* 'masculine' to be competing with women. But on the other hand, based on her *gender identity* as a woman she was (perhaps) *too* 'feminine' to be competing with men. Consequently, some might say that she had an unfair advantage competing with women. On the other hand, one might say that she would have had an unfair *dis*advantage if she had been 'forced' to compete with men. In fact, if we acknowledge the existence of a structurally based gender hierarchy – in which men (as a group) are superior to women (as a group) – it seems unfair to say that Stella Walsh did something wrong, that is, cheated.

Stella Walsh was, as a 'woman', subordinated to men in the gender hierarchy, which *may* mean that she had an initial disadvantage in sports.

Restricted to this aspect, she had no unfair advantage over other female athletes. It is as simple as that. Of course, this does not imply that she had no advantages at all. On the contrary, we have strong reason to believe that her genetic make-up meant that she had some advantages over most other female athletes. This is not controversial. Individual differences in genetic constitutions are not morally disturbing in themselves.

But to recognise individual differences in terms of genetic make-up is one thing; to separate athletes based on their sex/gender is a different thing.

Perhaps it is the *segregation* of sexes/genders that is the core problem. If it is, we may have good reasons to abolish sex-segregated sports. Or, as Torbjörn Tännsjö puts it:

> In sports it is crucial that the best person wins. Then sexual differences are simply irrelevant. If a female athlete can perform better than a male athlete, this female athlete should be allowed to compete with, and beat, the male athlete. If she cannot beat a certain male athlete, so be it. If the competition was fair, she should be able to face that he was more talented. It is really as simple as that. Sexual discrimination within sports does not have any better rationale than sexual discrimination in any other fields of our lives. (Tännsjö 2000, 101)

Tännsjö's main concern is of course elite sports, where winning is more important than just participating, and where the gender differences are commonly described as most relevant. His argument is quite convincing.

Because why should we accept sexual or gender discrimination within sports if we do not accept it elsewhere? The only reasonable argument in favour of such discrimination would be to say that the sex/gender discrimination in sport support fair competitions overall. But this argument suggests that we always should consider fairness before other moral values, and that sex/gender discrimination is not a part of the concept of fairness as a whole. All things considered, it seems problematic to support discrimination based on sex/gender if we simultaneously value fairness as something good.

Are we facing a conflict here? It is possible. The most obvious counter-argument would be that sex/gender-integrated competitions would promote unfairness. Such an argument presupposes that sex/gender should not only be considered in sports, but also that sex/gender should be considered as *directly* relevant in sports.

This does not mean that there are no differences at all that should be counted for; because there are. In sports such as wrestling and boxing, body weight plays a direct role in the outcome of the competitions. Therefore, we can easily accept weight classes in these sports. But different weight classes do not reinforce gender differences. Classifications based on sex/gender do.

This does not imply that there are no sex/gender differences to consider. For example, in absolute terms women's strength is approximately 50–60 per cent of men's strength in the upper body and 70–80 per cent of men's strength in the lower body (Koivula 1999, 11). But these differences do not have to have biological reasons. Nathalie Koivula argues: 'The smaller difference in strength for the lower body than the upper body can not be explained by differences in muscle physiology. The explanation can instead be found in social factors' (ibid.).

Now, women are not in general encouraged to be 'like men', and sports is in many ways shaped by men and 'for men'. This can mean that, if women are expected to be the 'weaker' sex/gender, it *makes* them 'weaker'.

Of course, one might argue that it does not matter whether female athletes in general are inferior to male athletes based on genetics or social circumstances. It is enough to say that they are inferior. And if they are, it seems unfair to force them to compete with male athletes.

Now, I believe it to be true that male athletes *as a group* perform 'better' in sports than female athletes *as a group – on average*, that is. If men and women would be competing against each other in (most) elite sports, men would most certainly win most of the time. This may be statistically true, but it is not obvious that the reason for such gender-nequal outcomes is based on biological differences between men and women.

If men and women had equal chances, the situation could have been different. For instance, if men and women hade same amount of resources and encouragement and if there were not such a thing as sex/gender inequality or even a concept of sex/gender – then maybe the world of sport would have been different. In fact, it seems reasonable to believe that it would have been a totally different world overall.

But based on the fact that the world includes socially constructed inequalities between men and women, one has several possible strategies to follow in terms of making the world (of sports) less unequal.

The suggestions for making the sports world sex/gender equal have been many. I will now discuss such an example.

In her famous article 'Sex Equality in Sports', Jane English argues that everyone should have equal right to what she calls *basic benefits* in sports, for instance

> health, the self-respect to be gained by doing one's best, the cooperation to be learned from working with teammates and the incentive gained from having opponents, the 'character' of learning to be a good loser and a good winner, the chance to improve one's skills and learn to accept criticism – and just plain fun. (English 1995, 284–5)

I think most of us would agree to this proposal. There is more to English's theory.

In contrast to basic benefits, English also elaborates another concept of benefits, so called *scarce benefits*. Scarce benefits means for instance prizes and publicity. No one can claim a right to these, or as English bluntly puts it: 'not everyone can claim an equal right to receive fan mail or appear on television' (English 1995, 285). So, how does this affect the issue of gender equality in sports?

To begin with, it is quite easy to see that male athletes get more attention than female athletes, at least generally speaking. Do we have reason to complain about this unequal situation? Jane English believes that we should complain. Because even though we are speaking about relatively privileged athletes, there is something questionable about the actual inequality at stake. If we believe in equality, this should also imply parties among the privileged groups of society (for instance elite athletes). If we now think this is a compelling premise, and I assume for the sake of argument that it is, we have to ask how we should make the inequality less unequal. English has a suggestion. She constructs a theory of distributive justice, for which she proposes a model of distribution where 'proportional attainments for the major social groups, should be applied to the scarce benefits' (ibid.). Thereby she also rejects the idea of sex-integrated competitions. She argues:

> The justification of maintaining separate teams for the sexes is the impact on women that integration would have. When there are virtually no female athletic stars, or when women receive much less prize money than men do, this is damaging to the self-respect of all women. Members of disadvantaged groups identify strongly with each other's success and failures. If women do not attain roughly equal fame and fortune in sports, it leads both men and women to think of women as naturally inferior. Thus, it is not a right of women tennis stars to the scarce benefits, but rather a right of all women to self-respect that justifies their demand for equal press coverage and prize money. (English 1995, 286)

English applies a traditional principle of equality of opportunity to sports, in much the same way as the principle is supposed to work as an instrument of favouring socially disadvantaged groups of society in other areas as well. In a sports context, it means for instance that a society is just only if the percentage of a 'major social group' corresponds to the population as a whole, which means that society is unjust if not half of professional athletes are women.

English identifies some obstacles for making this happen, though. For example, that sport mostly is based on male-specific physiological traits. She argues:

> In recent years, women have been making impressive progress in narrowing the gap between male and female performance. But there are apparently some *permanent* biological differences that affirmative action and consciousness raising will never change: women are smaller than men, they have a higher percentage of fat, they lack the hormones necessary for massive muscle development, they have a different hip structure and a slower oxygenation rate. (Ibid., emphasis added)

English's argument is problematic. It is, for instance, not uncommon that 'biological' arguments are used to legitimate the gender hierarchy, for example by seeing women's 'gender roles' as something that is 'natural' (Moller Okin 1979, 106). English falls into that pitfall when she refers to 'permanent biological differences' between men and women. Her position on this issue raises some questions. Can we be certain that the biological differences are permanent (for all time), and can we know for sure that biological differences are 'biological' and not social? And if so, why should we accept this 'matter of fact' as permanent? Is it even possible to determine a person's sex without having an idea of quite stable gender categories? What we here have to consider is that it may be extremely difficult to determine a person's sex from his or her social gender (Fausto-Sterling 1985). In other words, sex can be influenced by social factors. So which factors are relevant to a person's 'biological' sex? Is it the chromosomes, the genitalia or the gender? And what should be defined as a person's sex if the person's chromosomes do not correspond to his or her gender identity? In short, what should count?

However, English's solution to the gender inequality problem is a 'calling for development of new sports' (English 1995, 287). The reason for this is that the concept of sport (as we know it) 'contains a male bias' (ibid., 286 – 7). In short, society should interfere with the sports market mechanisms so that sports are better suited for female athletes (presumably with 'female' characteristics). In some way she makes a strong feminist case, if only in that she sees that another world is possible. Nonetheless, her proposal is problematic. In focusing on *female* characteristics, whether they are biologically or socially constructed, she creates an image of women as *the others*, the exception. In fact, her proposal may confirm what many critics of gender equality in sport (and elsewhere) would use as a weapon to fight gender equality as well as feminism. Besides, her proposal suggests that sport (as we know it) is better suited for 'male' physiology, which in itself seem rather biased.

English's proposal does not exist in an ideological vacuum. It can be traced to a specific kind of feminist analysis, radical feminism. One of the philosophical engineers of radical feminism, Catharine MacKinnon, defines radical feminism in a sports context in the following way:

> Radical feminism is not satisfied with women emulating the existing image of the athlete, which has been a male image. Neither with that, nor with the separate and vicarious role of cheerleader, not with other feminine physical pursuits that have been left to us. Instead, feminism moves to transform the meaning of athletics, of sport itself. (MacKinnon 2003, 268)

MacKinnon focuses quite hard on the often sexist gender stereotyping connected to sporting bodies. She also argues that it is not the gender differentiation that is the problem, but the gender hierarchy in which gender differentiation 'is only a strategy' (ibid.).

I fully agree with her that sexism hurts men and women in unequal ways, based on the gender inequality in society as a whole (ibid.). This far I follow her reasoning. But when she claims that it is *not* the *differentiation* in itself that is the problem, I stop following her.

I think we have reason to believe that it is the differentiation in itself that is the core problem. Without the differentiation there would not have been a gender hierarchy, and it is the gender differentiation that separates female bodies from male bodies. This objection does not undermine the logic within her theory, and MacKinnon's strategic proposal for gender equality presupposes a well-defined distinction between men and women. She writes: 'The place of women's athletics in a larger feminist analysis is that women *as women* have a survival stake in reclaiming our bodies in our physical relations with other people' (MacKinnon 2003, 270). Later on she continues that she thinks that women's physicality has a 'distinct meaning' through their bodies. The 'meaning' she speaks of, comes from women's oppression through their bodies. Based on this, women have 'something to offer the world of athletics', much as sport has something to offer women (ibid., 271). Does MacKinnon's suggestion offer a solution for liberating women in sports? I fail to see that.

Again, MacKinnon argues from a point of view where categories such as 'men' and 'women' are grounded in the very experiences of belonging to one of these two sexes (or genders). For MacKinnon this has a specific impact for her theory. It means, for example, that the oppression of women is based on the *experience* of being women in the patriarchal society. Her analytical strategy for making her point is to look at the sex/gender structure the same way as Marxists look at the structure of class.

According to orthodox Marxism, society is built on the basic opposition between capitalists and workers. Translated into MacKinnon's understanding of radical feminism, it means that the basic opposition in society is between men (as a group) and women (as a group). In Marxist theory workers are being 'robbed' of their labour (or fruits of their labour); in radical feminist theory women are being 'robbed' of their sexuality. The Marxist theory and MacKinnon's understanding of radical feminism are both theories in which power inequalities are at heart – but in quite different ways.

Women are socialised into this closed patriarchal structure, MacKinnon says. Therefore, she continues, the origin of 'woman' is constituted by another's (that is, men's) desire. Hence women are not autonomous. In fact, they do not even exist outside this structure, because outside this structure there is nothing.

Because MacKinnon believes that the basic opposition in society is between men and women, she draws the conclusion that every woman shares the same experience of being oppressed with other women. Therefore, she claims, is there a 'unity of women', where women's identity is founded upon the experience of being women (MacKinnon 1982).

Obviously, in her theory there is not much room for differences based on other factors than sex/gender. For that, her radical theory of experience has been criticised by other feminist theorists. Donna Haraway, for example, claims that MacKinnon's theory 'is a totalisation producing what Western patriarchy itself never succeeded in doing – feminists' consciousness of the non-existence of women, except as products of men's desire' (Haraway 1991, 159). I believe Haraway makes a compelling point here. Because following MacKinnon's theory to the end would probably lead to the conclusion that women should reinforce their 'femaleness' or 'womanhood'. But that would probably not serve women's status in sport. Separation cannot be the solution as long as the norms in society are based on masculine ideologies. Therefore we have strong reasons to reject her solution, even though it is easy from a feminist point of view to agree to her analysis of the state of society.

In other words, MacKinnon's theory does not serve as a sufficiently sharp tool against sex/gender discrimination in sports. On the contrary, I think her theory in practice would be counterproductive, in that it suggests reinforcement of already well-grounded stereotypes created in the sports context as such. So if we are not convinced that MacKinnon's arguments are sufficiently strong for making the world of sports less unequal, there might be better theoretical suggestions. If we want to obliterate sexism and gender discrimination in sports, we probably have to find ways of changing the focus from sporting gender-differentiated bodies to the sporting performances in themselves. Based on that, it may seem even stranger that radical feminists such as MacKinnon support sex/gender-segregated sports.

In conclusion, MacKinnon's arguments for gender equality do not threaten the gender hierarchy that radical feminists rightfully complain about. In fact, it seems rather sex/gender conservative to say that sex/gender is an *essential* quality that should count in sports. Rather, the problem is that sports produces (and re-produces) sex/gender as such.

But which is the best way of understanding this distinction between sex and gender?

The Myth of Natural Bodies: A Deconstruction of Sex and Gender in Sport

The debate among gender theorists about how to understand the sex/gender distinction has been going on ever since the distinction was first presented in the 1950s by the psychoanalyst Robert Stoller. Stoller invented the distinction when he studied the situation of transsexuals and found that there was not a correspondence between their ('biological') sex belonging and their gender identity. He also noted that their gender identities were much stronger than their connections to their (biological) sex (Gothlin 1999, 3). This seems reasonable. An identity is conceptually connected to what a person *is*. Of course, this does not imply that we know what the concept of *self* stands on. Perhaps the idea of having a self is built on a myth, but that does not mean that the myth does not have an impact on how we see ourselves as consciousness persons.

As I claimed earlier, it seems as if Stella Walsh fell between the concept of sex and the concept of gender. There was no correspondence between her 'biological' sex and her social gender. Therefore, she was a hybrid in sports. She was a 'natural' hybrid, according to our culture's definitions on sex and gender.

The sex/gender distinction has been elaborated from many angles. Probably the most far-reaching theories are formulated by poststructuralists such as the queer theorist Judith Butler.

Butler (1990, 7) argues that sex is 'as culturally constructed as gender'. The target of her critique is the idea that 'sex' is to be equivalent to what is supposed to be 'biological', 'natural', 'body', 'stable' et cetera, whereas 'gender' is supposed to be equivalent to what is 'political', 'cultural', 'mind', 'unstable' et cetera.

Poststructuralists 'are *unhappy* with these dichotomies' (Moi 1999, 34). The point is that the concept of sex can very well change when it is put in the light of gender structures or hierarchies. Considering historical, social and cultural differences in gender, we have reasons to believe that the concept of gender (as well as the concept of sex) is something rather unstable. But this does not imply that social determinism is a much better alternative. In fact, the rejection of biological determinism does not rescue us from being prisoners in the 'gender war'. Or, as Toril Moi (1999, 38) chooses to put it, social determinism 'is nothing but biological determinism with a liberal face'. And she continues: 'Even if we all agreed to have five sexes...nothing guarantees that we would get more than two genders, or that we wouldn't be stuck with five sets of oppressive gender norms instead of two' (ibid.). Based on this, one can argue that the concept of gender and the gender norms in themselves do not have to be more 'liberating' than being stuck with 'biological' norms.

However, concepts such as 'man' and 'woman' may be 'blurred at the edges', but it does not mean that they are 'meaningless or useless', Moi argues (ibid., 39). In reference to the Wittgensteinian argument considering the concept 'game' – which says that a blurred concept can still be a concept – Moi argues: '[H]ermaphroditism, transvestism, transsexuality, and so on show up the fuzziness at the edges of sexual difference, but the concepts of "man" and "woman" or the opposition between them are not thereby threatened by disintegration' (ibid.).

Moi's point is that the deconstruction of the sex/gender distinction does not get rid of the problems that come with the concepts in themselves. Therefore she and others – for example Heinämaa (1997) – argue that the concept of gender should be eliminated. A deconstruction of the sex/gender distinction is not sufficient, nor is it sufficient to 'kill' the concept of sex as Judith Butler suggests. I agree with Moi in this sense.

Because, in using the concept of gender, we have not eliminated how bodies are differentiated into 'masculine' and 'feminine' bodies (see for example Rubin 1975). And the discourse of 'masculine' and 'feminine' bodies works within the sex/gender distinction; either we define bodies from 'biological' perspectives or from 'social' perspectives.

Based on this premise, one can – as Moi claims – argue that it is useful not to speak about sex and gender but about 'body' and 'subjectivity'; because the 'relationship between body and subjectivity is neither necessary nor arbitrary, but contingent' (Moi 1999, 114). To this argument one can add that the concept of gender may recreate old-fashioned 'gender roles'. In a sports context this has a special significance, simply because of the strong masculinity norms present in the field. The story of Stella Walsh has shown us this.

However, Walsh is not the only one in the history of sport suspected of 'cheating' based on different ideological views on sex/gender.

Transgendered persons, for example, have always 'caused' problems for sports organisations. The growing awareness of the concept of transgender has in fact 'forced' sports organisations to make ethically controversial decisions. An example of that can be dated to 2004, when the Medical Commission of the IOC decided that transsexual athletes should be allowed to compete in the Olympic Games in Athens the same year; even though transsexuals have always had that right. But by the acknowledgment of this 'group' of people, the IOC thought it would have to have special rules to control them. The decision made by the medical commission sharpened the control over transgendered persons.

The incentive for making special rules to control transgendered athletes came after the Danish-Australian golf player Mianne Bagger's sex change from man to woman in 1995. At that time, golf organisations such as the European Ladies' Professional Golf Association and the Ladies European Tour (LET) denied her access to their competitions. The Swedish golf association, on the other hand, took a different approach. It allowed her to play in competitions it arranged. The IOC also took her side. Still, the question of transgendered athletes landed on the sports agenda.

Obviously, the powerful sports organisations felt they had to decide something regarding this matter. Arne Ljungqvist, the president of the IOC Medical Commission, said in an interview: 'In the world of sports, we must have special rules, and we have such rules now. For instance, [for transgendered persons] there must be a transition period for two years' (Söderberg 2004, 23 – my translation). The rules proclaim, for instance, that 'male' transsexuals have to have their gonads removed if they are allowed to compete. By removing their gonads they will presumably be 'weaker'. Even though Ljungqvist also says that the focus on muscle mass is overrated, the decision is made within a biological discourse. This may all seem rather uncontroversial. But it is not. In fact, the decision is highly sexist!

I do not think it would have been possible to make such a decision, or to create 'special rules' for transgendered athletes, without the sexist stereotype of 'women' being the 'weaker sex'. The IOC's decision substantiates that stereotype. Also, the IOC's (discriminatory) decision is an example of the fact that every athlete *has to be* either a 'man' or a 'woman'. One can argue that this does not make the world of sports any different from other contexts. But the consequences can be different.

For instance, those who undergo a sex change are not allowed to compete – that is, perform their profession – for two years; this of course is especially harsh when it comes to athletes, who generally have rather short careers. But this is not the only ethically objectionable consequence.

The enforcement of (only) two gender categories, 'men' and 'women', makes the importance of sex/gender verification tests valid. Of course, this is also a highly controversial issue.

Since the year 2000 sex/gender verification tests are not allowed. The abandonment of such tests came after strong protests from female athletes who had found them offensive and sexist. On the other hand, there are other ways of verifying an individual's sex/gender. The intense use of advanced doping tests can perhaps be seen as an alternative to the former sex/gender verification tests (Skirstad 2000, 119). This obviously means that doping testing is an instrument of discipline, placing athletes into very specific and culturally defined gender categories.

The Heart of Sports Culture: Masculinity Norms and Gender Discipline

Tara Magdalinski and Karen Brooks state that 'Modern sport has always been firmly linked to a patriarchal project that seeks to establish and maintain strict cultural boundaries that police what is feminine and what is masculine' (Magdalinski and Brooks 2002, 209). Obviously, I agree with this (well documented) statement. Because can we imagine sport (as we know it) without its gender constructions? I think it would be difficult. And as long as we elaborate the concepts of 'masculinity' and 'femininity' – concepts we use to differentiate women from men in terms of bodily functions, physiological traits and performances – it may be difficult to reach gender equality in sports, because of the cultural connotations that lie within these concepts.

At the same time, we also seem to focus quite hard on the connection between a person's 'sex' and supposed gender. Consider, for example, figure skating. According to the Olympic Games rules for pairs figure skating and ice dancing, two men or two women are not allowed to compete as a couple. (In the Gay Games they are, though.) Suppose it would have been allowed, would it then serve the idea of gender equality? Of course it would have been better compared to the original situation.

Nonetheless, pairs figure skating and ice dancing are about competing in accordance with certain norms, norms based on ideas on masculinity and femininity. This in itself has nothing to do with the skaters' sex, even if it is believed to be so. In short, it is the gender norms of masculinity and femininity that are in focus in these sports.

Are there any alternative gender patterns to consider? What happens if we mix masculinity and femininity? The concept of *androgyny* may be such an alternative. The concept is considered to be a mixture of masculinity and femininity characteristics (Connell 2002, 34). But, I would say, the concept of androgyny is not satisfying either, because it contains the concepts of masculinity and femininity. Therefore we still have to work with concepts that divide bodies into these two categories.

Each category contains a certain set of culturally defined qualities. Usually, we associate 'masculine' qualities with muscle strength while 'feminine' qualities are associated with, for example, cooperation and sensitivity (Tännsjö 2000, 109).

The division on this account is not satisfying from a gender egalitarian perspective; even if, as for example Tännsjö suggests, 'feminine' qualities 'should not only be added to existing qualities but, in many cases, be exchanged for existing qualities' (ibid., 109 – 10).

The problem with this proposal is that it does not challenge gender-based stereotypes. Instead there is a risk of confirming and perhaps even strengthening them. In fact, one can argue that the concept of masculinity and femininity is an example of how something can be disciplined by using the concept of gender overall, given that masculinity/femininity norms discipline people (as I believe they do). Often, femininity becomes the exception except in sports where 'female' qualities are appreciated (as for instance in *female* figure skating).

Such exceptions do not undermine the masculine *sports culture*, though. Sports culture still is heavily gendered as a masculine phenomenon.

I believe we have no reason not to think that sport plays a significant role in the everyday constructions of gender stereotypes. Or, as the gender theorist R.W. Connell describes it:

> In historically recent times, sport has come to be the leading definer of masculinity in mass culture. Sport provides a continuous display of men's bodies in motion. Elaborate and carefully monitored rules bring these bodies into stylized contests with each other. In these contests a combination of superior force (provided by size, fitness, teamwork) and superior skill (provided by planning, practice and intuition) will enable one side to win. (Connell 1995, 54)

The kind of masculinity Connell describes gives us a picture of the gender hierarchy that every man and woman has to relate to, and which also excludes women from sport. Connell says:

> The institutional organization of sport embeds definite social relations: competition and hierarchy among men, exclusion or domination of women. These social relations of gender are both realized and symbolized in the bodily performances. Thus men's greater sporting prowess has become a theme of backlash against feminism. It serves as symbolic proof of men's superiority and right to rule. (Ibid.)

Sport may very well serve as an example of 'hegemonic masculinity' (Connell 1995, 76ff.). Perhaps one way of breaking this hegemony would be to include women in the symbolic language and institutions of sport. Iris Marion Young (1995, 265) even claims that it is even 'necessary' to 'humanize' sports. She continues:

> Mere inclusion of women in the existing concept and institutions of sport, however, is not sufficient. Sports programs for women today frequently model themselves on and measure themselves by the standards of sport programs which have traditionally been reserved for men. There is more justice in this situation than in the exclusion of women entirely, but the masculinist bias of sport is not thereby removed. (Young 1995, 265)

Young describes a situation where the gender hierarchy favours men, based on the fact that sports are masculine by habit and tradition. Consequently, the gender discrimination is institutionalised. Now, can we imagine that advanced medical and/or gene technologies will make a difference in this particular sense, which is to make sports gender-equal or gender-neutral?

Athletic Enhancement Technologies and the Gender Equality Issue

Can new technology give us tools for breaking down the gates of the 'gender prison'? Or, will it lead to a situation where the already strong masculine norms in sport will be strengthened? This question can be put in another way: *Is there a conflict between athletic enhancement technologies and gender equality?* There might be. But if we think there is such a contradiction we also have to understand the analytical reason for making such an assumption. To say that there is a *conceptual* contradiction would be strange. But sports are not all about concepts; they are also about conceptions of gender. In fact, I think it is difficult to watch sport without watching gender. And gender issues are often (or always) about power. Which body is the most valuable one in terms of sport? Which gender?

But even if we do not see a conceptual contradiction between athletic enhancement technologies and gender equality, we certainly have to see the gender inequality that lies within the history of all societies and in the conceptions of gender and sport. We should not take this issue lightly, as long as we see ourselves as egalitarians (which I assume that we do in some sense of the word). But, the concept of equality and the concept of gender equality are theoretically problematic. Again, is there a way out of the 'gender prison' we have created for ourselves?

Applied to sports technology, we have reason to raise the question whether technology in general, and medical and/or gene technology especially, can be an instrument in favour of gender equality and/or gender neutralism. One can, for instance, claim that medicine appears to legitimate, rather than challenge, the existing gender order.

It is not a secret that technologies, and especially medical, reproductive and gene technologies, often lead to serious ethical controversies. Not least among feminist theorists, there has always been a well-founded criticism of technological innovations. The main reason for that is simply that women have often been exploited by, and have been merely objects for, male scientists. For example, when it comes to reproductive technologies it has always been men who have had control over the technological means of reproduction. Historically, and symbolically as well as in practice, women have been more vulnerable than men to being exploited, as a result of the gender hierarchy. Solely based on that, many feminists find it problematic to say that medical technology would promote women's liberation (see for example Dworkin 1983; Rowland 1984, 356 – 71; Katz Rothman 1984, 23 – 35; Corea 1988). The feminist critics are many, but there also exist feminist advocates. For example, the radical feminist Shulamith Firestone, who suggests *ectogenesis* (that is pregnancy outside the womb) in order to liberate women from 'the tyranny of reproduction' (Firestone 2002, 185).

The controversy among feminists reminds us that one can have more than one feminist view on this issue. As implied, usually the debate concerns reproduction, for example abortion, insemination, in-vitro fertilisation, surrogate motherhood and cloning. Some of the feminists welcome new technologies, based on principles of autonomy, while others think that new technologies restrain autonomy in becoming just another instrument for male scientists and doctors to dominate women. These kinds of controversies exist also when it comes to advanced sport technologies, including genetic modification in sport.

Usually, genetic modification, or 'gene-doping', is described as a more advanced form of doping. But, as Andy Miah argues, 'Ethical arguments against doping in sport do not have the same force when applied to genetic modification. Moreover, it would be a mistake to categorise genetic enhancement as merely another form of doping, since it is a conceptually and culturally different kind of technology' (Miah 2004, 160). To this one can add that genetic modification technologies may also have an impact on gender constructions. From a gender egalitarian view, Claudio Tamburrini and Torbjörn Tännsjö welcome the promises of what they call 'Bio-Amazons', that is, genetically designed female athletes as something supposed to serve equality in sports. Considering the issue of male norms in sport, they argue:

> Who says muscles and raw strength are exclusively masculine attributes? Male physical strength is no doubt a direct result of biological factors. But are not these biological factors themselves also the result of the evolutionary history of mankind? How do we know, say, which level of testosterone males at present would have if societies had adopted more equal gender roles in the past? (Tamburrini and Tännsjö 2005, 192)

Later on, they continue: '[I]f some women decide that they want to become as strong as the strongest men, why should they not be allowed to do as they see fit?' (Ibid.)

Tamburrini and Tännsjö make a strong case in favour of gender equality. Bio-Amazons, they say, 'will contribute to a fairer sports world, in two senses: by allowing (at least some) women to attain rewards and benefits until now exclusively enjoyed by males, and by equalising conditions between them and transsexual athletes' (ibid.). Tamburrini's and Tännsjö's support for Bio-Amazons have been criticised for different reasons.

Susan Sherwin and Meredith Schwartz, for instance, argue that 'they quickly collapse any distinction between same treatment and equal treatment.... We ... believe that it is a mistake to interpret equality as sameness' (Sherwin and Schwartz 2005, 200). Other critics, such as Simona Giordano and John Harris, believe that Tamburrini's and Tännsjö's suggestion hide a male chauvinist ideology. In fact, they think that gender differences *should not* be corrected, and they continue:

> It seems to us that the facts that there are male and female sports and exercise activities is in no way discriminatory or an offence to equality. People can still and should still be treated with equal concern and respect regardless of the tournaments in which they participate, regardless of their physical differences or genetic structure. Gender, and what it entails in terms of physical capacities, is not an element that requires medical or genetic remedy. In so far as gender constitutes 'a disadvantage' in some contexts this is purely a contingent matter. It is, in short, a social, political, economic and moral problem requiring social, political, economic and moral solutions. To offer a medical or genetic solution exacerbates the problem and insults women. (Giordano and Harris 2005, 216)

The provocative idea of Bio-Amazon programming and the objections against that idea say much about the internal problems that come with the sex/gender distinction.

Both views seem to be based on the 'necessity' of the concept of gender. I will develop this issue later.

For now, let me just state that sport in general promotes gender differentiation, and sex/gender-segregated sports probably recreate traditional gender patterns. One can even argue that sport (as we know it) in itself holds a 'male chauvinist ideology'. On this account alone, it is not, or should not be, particularly radical to say that women should have the right to become as strong as their male colleagues in sport. In other words, it really should not be a problem if female athletes become more 'like men' (whatever that is).

But suppose that the consequence would be that only women – and not men – would be 'forced' to manipulate their bodies in order to become 'as strong as the strongest men', as Tamburrini and Tännsjö put it. Would that be a problem? To be clear and fair, Tamburrini and Tännsjö do not suggest that only women should have the right to genetically manipulate their bodies. Also men should have the right to transcend the sex/gender boundaries. Although their argument works in favour of the idea of individuals crossing sex/gender barriers, it still entails the acceptance of the concept of gender, and the concept of gender differentiates bodies into certain (gender) norms, and that involves and promotes (gender) discrimination. Perhaps we have come to a dead end.

In fact, it is not obvious at all that medical technology will challenge the traditional gender constructions. On the contrary, many of them probably serve as instruments for maintaining very specific gender norms.

Cosmetic surgery is an obvious example of that. People who use cosmetic surgery are usually following very specific cultural norms. In turning bodies into symbolic capital, they follow the Western manuscript closely. In practice it usually means that women use cosmetic surgery (and other medical technologies) to become more 'feminine' whereas men use cosmetic surgery (and other medical technologies) to become more 'masculine', often based on Western, middle-class, white norms (Sandell 2003, 189 – 213). At the same time, undergoing cosmetic surgery can be seen as a form of individual strategy, in order to improve chances of success in life. Why would medical technology in sport be any different or upsetting?

It is, of course, not certain that medical technology has to serve the existing gender order. We are not speaking of 'natural laws' here. Quite the opposite; one can imagine that the use of medical technology can serve as a 'disturbing' instrument towards the gender constructions of today.

Now the technologisation of the human has become been more and more advanced. Some would say that the next step on the technological journey would be the full creation of so-called cyborgs, simply described as 'symbiotic fusions of organic life and technological systems' (Davis-Floyd and Dumit 1998, 1). An even more simple description would be that cyborgs are a hybrid of 'human beings' and 'machines'. Perhaps the cyborg (monster) can rescue us from the gender inequality we face within (and outside) the sports context? There we also enter another moral minefield.

Monsters of Sport and the Promises of Cyborg Athletes: The Death of Sport (As We Know It)?

One can read the story of Stella Walsh as a moral story of a person who (unintentionally or not) acted against the Western view of sex and gender. She is not the only one doing that.

There have been many of them in sports history. For example, the runner Jarmila Kratochvílová from Czechoslovakia (today the Czech Republic), who beat the world record at 800 metres for women in 1983. (She is still the world record holder on that distance.) She was constantly suspected of using illegal performance-enhancing drugs. In the media she was referred to as 'the third sex'. Both Walsh and Kratochvílová diverged from the traditional gender norms. In that sense they become 'monsters' of sport. And the 'monster' as a metaphor plays an important role in Western thought. In her classical article 'A Cyborg Manifesto: Science, Technology, and Socialist-Feminism in the Late Twentieth Century', Donna Haraway says:

> Monsters have always defined the limits of community in Western imaginations. The Centaurs and Amazons of ancient Greece established the limits of the centred polis of the Greek male human by their disruption of marriage and boundary pollutions of the warrior with animality and woman. Unseparated twins and hermaphrodites were the confused human material in early modern France who grounded discourse on the natural and supernatural, medical and legal, portents and diseases – all crucial to establishing modern identity. The evolutionary and behavioural sciences of monkeys and apes have marked the multiple boundaries of late twentieth-century industrial identities. Cyborg monsters in feminist science fiction define quite different political possibilities and limits from those proposed by the mundane fiction of Man and Woman. (Haraway 1991, 180)

Following Haraway's short odyssey through the mythological and historical background and understanding of the concept of monster, one can say that it was Walsh's and Kratochvílová's masculine bodies that made them 'monstrous'. Similar 'accusations' were directed at the female athletes from East Germany when they dominated especially swimming and the athletics during the 1970s and 1980s.

It is not a secret that they were taking performance-enhancing drugs. Many spoke of these athletes as 'manufactured' in state-controlled doping laboratories. Obviously, these (female) athletes not only challenged 'impossible' results, but also the image of what a 'woman' *is* or *should be*.

Of course, there is an important difference between the athletes from East Germany and for instance Stella Walsh. Walsh did not have access to advanced medical technology. She was just born with a certain set of genes which helped her to be a great runner.

So is there a moral difference between the 'manufactured' East German athletes of the 1970s and 1980s and Walsh? Of course, one can easily argue that the East German sports culture produced athletes by intentionally using medical technology in order to gain (unfair) advantages in the international sports competitions. Both Walsh and the female athletes of East Germany challenged certain gender norms. But does it mean that they challenged the gender constructions as such? I think it would be too far-fetched to make such a claim.

Is there a solution to this complex issue? Maybe there is. But first we may have to enter another theory of sport technology: cyborg (feminist) athletism, where the concept of sex and the concept of gender are eliminated once and for all. What the consequences may be of such a theory is open for philosophical speculation. Perhaps it may lead to the death of sport (as we know it), if we consider sport in itself to be gendered. Another possibility is to say that sport without gender makes sport and sport performances more 'genuine' or 'pure'. This possibility would perhaps imply that cyborgs are the 'saviours' of (future) sport, or at least only an integrated part of the logic of sports and sports culture. Some may reply that this speculative suggestion is to stretch this issue too far. Still, I think it is a theoretical possibility worth considering. I guess it all depends on what we think of the concept of cyborgs as such.

According to Donna Haraway's cyborg theory, cyborgs are considered to be 'self-moving, self-designing, autonomous' (Haraway 1991, 152). In her 'manifesto', Haraway develops a feminist cyborg theory in which she makes the following proclamation:

> This chapter is an argument for *pleasure* in the confusion of boundaries and for *responsibility* in their construction. It is also an effort to contribute to socialist-feminist culture and theory in a postmodernist, non-naturalist mode and in the utopian tradition of imagining a world without gender, which is perhaps a world without genesis, but maybe also a world without end. (Ibid., 150)

According to Haraway's cyborg mythology, the cyborg challenges every known dichotomy in Western tradition, for example, self/other, mind/body, culture/nature and male/female. These and others dichotomies 'have all been systematic to the logics and practices of domination of women, people of colour, nature, workers, animals – in short, domination of all constituted as others, whose task is to mirror the self' (ibid., 177). But, Haraway continues, 'High-tech culture challenges these dualisms in intriguing ways. It is not clear who makes and who is made in the relation between human and machine.'

The cyborg 'is a creature in a post-gender world', Haraway says (ibid., 150). Are we there yet? I think many of us would answer no, we are not. But perhaps we are, we just do not want to see it that way. Maybe because most of us still believe in the distinction between 'reality' and 'fiction'. Perhaps it is about time to 'think again'.

Usually, I believe we think of cyborgs only in terms of characters taken from science-fiction literature and science-fiction movies. We may think of Mary Shelley's *Frankenstein*'s 'monster' or James Cameron's *Terminator*. Are they 'good' role models or ambassadors for the cyborgs? Donna Haraway would answer no. They are not. In fact, we can question if they should be considered as cyborgs at all.

They are, for example, (heavily) gendered in that they are constructed in accordance with very traditional masculinity norms: they are, for instance, taller and more muscular and 'stronger' than the average (male) person. In other words, they are portrayed as 'enhanced' male persons. Consider, for example, the masculine techno-body of Arnold Schwarzenegger (who plays the character Terminator). It is a body of a 'machine-enhanced warrior' (Haraway 1995, xii).

Neither Frankenstein's monstrous creation in Shelley's novel, nor Terminator challenge the fundamental dichotomies in Western thought, including the dichotomy between the concepts 'male' and 'female' (Haraway 1991, 177). They confirm them!

Still, Frankenstein's 'monster' as well as Terminator are popular images of cyborgs in popular culture. They both serve to create a distance between 'humans' and 'machines'. And based on the 'fact' that we are humans, cyborgs are 'the Others'.

But let us now leave the images from the popular culture aside, and instead focus on the *concept* of the cyborg, and connect the concept to 'reality'.

The 'boundary between science fiction and social reality is an optical illusion', says Haraway (1991, 177). And she continues: 'By the late twentieth century, our time, a mythic time, we are all chimeras, theorized and fabricated hybrids of machine and organism; in short, we are cyborgs. The cyborg is our ontology; it gives us our politics. The cyborg is a condensed image of both imagination and material reality (ibid., 150).

Still, to most of us, cyborgs belong to the future and not to the present. Cyborgs are *fiction* and not *reality*. And we do not consider cyborgs to have an identity as cyborgs. But the harder it gets to distinguish between humans and machines, the harder it will be not to recognise cyborg identities, I presume. As a matter of fact, modern medicine, for instance, 'is full . . . of cyborgs', Haraway claims (ibid.). This may be true, only in that it has become increasingly harder to separate the 'natural' from the 'artificial' within the context of medicine and science in general. More important, it seems that modern society strives to escape what is considered to be 'natural' (and that for good reasons).

It seems already difficult, if not impossible, to draw a clear line between what is 'natural' and what is 'artificial'; it may even be difficult to make a distinction between 'natural' and 'artificial' persons in some sense. If we consider this to be reasonable, we will also find it difficult to draw a clear line between *natural born 'cheaters'* and *artificially constructed 'cheaters'*. Or, in other words, in terms of *personal identities* it may be difficult to see any relevant difference between someone who is born with a certain set of genes, which is to his or her advantage, and a person who has been medically or genetically modified.

Considering the latter example, we can notice two sorts of genetic modification: *somatic genetic modification* and *germ-line genetic modification* (Munthe 2000). In the former type of modification, the genetic interventions are implemented in already existing persons, and in the latter type of modification, the genetic interventions are implemented on embryos. Regardless of technique, one can consider the result as something that becomes a part of that person's identity.

What can this mean for the future of sports? And what does it mean in terms of sport ethics?

Suppose, for instance, that someone has manipulated an embryo by implementing artificial chromosomes. This person, when he/she/it grows up, will become an outstanding runner or swimmer. His/her/its 'natural'/'artificial' talents will be a part of his/her/its identity. Suppose we consider this person to be a cyborg. Should we exclude this person from official sports competitions? Or, should we embrace cyborg technologies that make this person to be an outstanding athlete? In other words, is there something morally upsetting about these technology? Probably not. Or, as James Hughes puts it:

> We have an ethical responsibility to help one another achieve our highest potentials, not just the current human average. The enhancement of ordinary to extraordinary abilities is as much a social good as the correction of a disability or illness. When we educate children we don't devote all our resources to kids performing below average because we also want the brighter kids to achieve as much as they can. We don't devote all our Olympic resources to the para-Olympics because we are also delighted to see how much the most talented can achieve. (Hughes 2004, 234)

Considering the quotation from Hughes, it is not evident (at all) that the 'cyborgisation' of humans challenges current ethical norms. So why even try to keep the division between 'humans' and 'machines' clear when it seems to be a lost game, not at least in a sports sphere? Or, as Andy Miah likes to put it:

> [S]port is already posthuman. Athletes have already metamorphosed into super-humans, blurred suitably by the softening presentation of modern television. Athletes are

ambassadors of transhumanism, placed at the cutting edge of human boundaries of capability. The athlete's body is in a state of flux, continually transcending itself, and thus perpetuating transhuman ideas about the biophysics of humanity. (Miah 2003)

At the same time it seems that the cyborg as we know him/her/it often represents an image of a masculine ideal. The examples of Frankenstein's monster and the movie character Terminator, for instance, seem to be more of caricatures of a 'masculinist reproductive dream' than a vision of a feminist cyborg ideal (Haraway 1991, 152).

So what is the point of cyborg athletics if we do not escape the gendered inequality problem? Perhaps there is a 'last straw' in this sense?

Perhaps we should not focus on the 'objective' physiological construction of the cyborg, but instead focus on the identity of the cyborg. Ted Butryn, for instance, discusses this issue in terms of 'self-technologization'. He argues:

> The female athlete who transgresses human-machine, as well as male-female, boundaries by taking steroids is not re-defining herself by conforming to some established criteria for a female athlete. Rather, she is affirming her unique identity through creatively employing *self* technologies, and in the process challenging traditional, often oppressive, notions of gender roles in sport. She has not sought to become 'more male', but rather to pursue authenticity by cyborgizing her body, despite what others (e.g. her fellow athletes, fans, and so on) may think. (Butryn 2002, 123)

I believe Butryn has a good point. The problem might be that the *self* is not obviously autonomous, in that it may well be constructed by circumstances beyond his/her/itself. Therefore, one may argue that the problem here is not the cyborgisation of bodies, or that cyborg bodies are shaped in certain ways, but that we tend to name the bodies according to certain gender norms. For example, when we speak about 'males' and 'females' we recreate these categories, and in doing so we also may recreate the conceptions hidden in these categories. And in the conceptions we may very well find a social and political constructed hierarchy. When we, for instance, speak of *women's rights*, we may construct women as 'the others'. On the other hand, from a strategic point of view, this may be politically motivated. (For instance, we may need 'groups' of some sort, if politically and economically oppressed individuals are to have a chance to improve their lives.) But it does not make us escape from the main problems that are hidden within the concepts as such.

In a sports context, organisations, media, fans and so on create or recreate boundaries among individuals, and sentence them to the 'gender prison'.

Cyborgs, whether they exist or not in reality, are still 'the others', the subversive 'monsters' who challenge 'traditional' masculine gendered sport ideals; if we do not consider them to be caricatures of the sport ideals, that is.

Cyborgs (and of course cyborg athletes) can be a result of 'natural' genetic mutations and/or 'artificial' genetic manipulation. Obviously, they confuse the boundaries between several popular dichotomies. Not allowing them to compete based on that would be a form of (genetic) discrimination.

Now if sports society (continues to) discriminate(s) against 'cyborgs', it is doing so on basis of the physiological traits and presumed identities of the cyborgs.

Therefore the discrimination against cyborgs can be considered to be as morally repulsive as discrimination based on sex/gender, 'race'/ethnicity, sexuality, (dis)ability, class etcetera.

Conclusion: Sports Without the Concept of Gender

I began this article by telling the story of Stella Walsh. Stella Walsh challenged the dichotomy between 'men' and 'women'. Her body was 'masculine' (that is, muscular). Her gender identity was as a 'woman'. Thereby she challenged the traditional 'gender roles'. Stella Walsh was subversive. As a 'masculine' woman she was a 'monster'.

What if her body had been a 'machine'? What if we all had bodies like machines? Would it make any difference? It is not obvious. By 'doing gender', one can easily make something that is at first gender-neutral into something that is (heavily) gendered.

Various things, things that initially have no gender, may be gendered for many reasons (for example, personal, political, ideological or commercial reasons). But what about bodies? Are bodies basically gender-neutral, but become gendered because of certain set of norms? I believe it to be so. Why should we otherwise connect masculinity to muscularity?

We consider muscularity to be masculine. And because sports are based on masculinity norms, it means that muscular sports bodies are the norm. Is there a way out of this masculinised sports culture?

Perhaps the theoretical solution comes with the cyborg, or the cyborg identity? Imagine not being able to see the difference between 'man' and 'machine'. Suppose we cannot see the difference between the technologies being used for athletic performances and the athletes themselves. The athlete has become the 'machine'. If so, it will become more and more difficult to see the difference between the 'natural' sporting bodies and the techniques that make the bodies perform. One can also imagine that the sporting activities become an integrated part of the athlete's identity. Still, the cyborg is 'subversive' in terms of Cartesian dualisms. Considering the interest among sports organisations especially of keeping the gates clear from 'monsters', they accept discrimination for the sake of 'equality' and 'fairness'.

What are they afraid of? One can only speculate. Perhaps they are afraid of losing control over their self-given right to define – *and therefore discriminate* – those who, for one reason or another, challenge the boundaries with their very bodies and identities; whether they are born with a certain set of genes or manipulated (medically or genetically) to be who they are or want to be.

But what is so fair about sport (as we know it), when it constantly entails gender discrimination? And what does it mean in terms of the future of sport? Can we imagine sport without gender, or would an elimination of gender become the death of sport (as we know it)? If so, would it be too hard to digest? One could for instance try imagining the development of a new and non-gendered sports culture different from the present. Maybe this seems too 'far out' or too much of 'science fiction'? I do not know. On the other hand, many things have been seen as 'science fiction' at first, and then become 'reality'. So why not?

However, with the ongoing development of so-called gene-doping and cyborg technology, we will perhaps face a future where sports (as we know it) occurs in its purest form; that is, where athletes get evaluated by their athletic performance only and not by their gender and where it becomes impossible to discriminate athletes based on their body constitution and gender identity. Some may say this suggestion is way too 'idealistic' or 'utopian'. Maybe it is.

But if we take the issue of (gender) equality seriously, we may also have to attack the heart of gender inequality or gender discrimination, and not just the symptoms or the effects of it.

And a morally reasonable way of meeting this issue is to say that the problem is *not* the individuals who (for one reason or another) transcend certain gender categories but the categories *in themselves*.

REFERENCES

BREIVIK, G. 2005. Sport, gene doping and ethics. In *Genetic Technology and Sport – Ethical Questions*, edited by C. Tamburrini and T. Tännsjö. London and New York: Routledge: 165 – 77.

BUTLER, J. 1990. *Gender Trouble. Feminism and the Subversion of Identity*. New York and London: Routledge.

BUTRYN, T. 2002. Cyborg horizons: Sport and the ethics of self-technologization. In *Sport Technology: History, Philosophy and Policy*, edited by A. Miah and S.B. Eassom. Amsterdam, Boston, MA, and London: Elsevier Science Ltd: 111 – 33.

CONNELL, R.W. 1995. *Masculinities*. Berkeley and Los Angeles, CA: University of California Press.

———. 2002. *Gender*. Cambridge: Polity.

COREA, G. 1988. *The Mother Machine. Reproductive Technologies from Artificial Insemination to Artificial Wombs*. London: The Women's Press.

DAVIS-FLOYD, R. and J. DUMIT. 1998. Cyborg babies. Children of the third millennium. In *Cyborg Babies. From Techno-Sex to Techno-Tots*, edited by R. Davis-Floyd and J. Dumit. New York and London: Routledge: 1 – 20.

DWORKIN, A. 1983. *Right-Wing Women. The Politics of Domesticated Females*. London: The Women's Press.

ENGLISH, J. 1995. Sex equality in sports. In *Philosophic Inquiry in Sport*, edited by W. Morgan and K. Meier. Champaign, IL: Human Kinetics: 284 – 8. This article was first published 1978 in *Philosophy & Public Affairs* 7 (3): 269 – 77.

FAUSTO-STERLING, A. 1985. *Myths of Gender. Biological Theories About Women and Men*. New York: Basic Books.

FIRESTONE, S. 2002. *The Dialectic of Sex. The Case for Feminist Revolution*. New York: Farrar, Strauss & Giroux (orig. pub. 1970).

GIORDANO, S. and J. HARRIS. What is gender equality in sports? In *Genetic Technology and Sport – Ethical Questions*, edited by C. Tamburrini and T. Tännsjö. London and New York: Routledge: 209 – 17.

GIULIANOTTI, R. 2005. *Sport. A critical sociology*. Cambridge: Polity.

GOTHLIN, E. 1999. *Kön eller genus* ['Sex or gender?'], Göteborg: Nationella sekretariatet för genusforskning.

HARAWAY, D. 1991. A cyborg manifesto: Science, technology, and socialist-feminism in the late twentieth century. In *Simians, Cyborgs, and Women: The Reinvention of Nature*. New York: Routledge.

———. 1995. Cyborgs and symbionts. Living together in the New World Order. In *The Cyborg Handbook*, edited by C. Hables. New York and London: Routledge: xi – xx.

HEINÄMAA, S. 1997. What is a woman? Butler and Beauvoir on the foundations of the sexual difference. *Hypatia. A journal of Feminist Philosophy* 12 (1): 20 – 40.

HUGHES, J. 2004. *Citizen Cyborg. Why Democratic Societies Must Respond to the Redesigned Human of the Future*. Cambridge, MA: Westview Press.

KATZ ROTHMAN, B. 1984. The meanings of choice in reproductive technology. In *Test-Tube Women. What Future for Motherhood?* edited by R. Arditti, R. Duelli Klein and S. Minden. London, Boston, MA, Melbourne and Henley: Pandora Press: 23–35.

KOIVULA, N. 1999. *Gender in Sport*. Stockholm: Department of Psychology, Stockholm University.

LARSSON, H. 2005. Queer idrott ['Queer sport']. In *Queersverige*, edited by D. Kulick, Stockholm: Natur och Kultur: 110–35.

LOLAND, S. 2002. *Fair Play in Sport. A Moral Norm System*. London and New York: Routledge.

MACKINNON, C. 1982. Feminism, Marxism, method, and the state: An agenda for theory. *Signs. Journal of Women in Culture and Society* 7 (31): 515–44.

———. 2003. Women, self-possession, and sport. In *Sport Ethics. An Anthology*, edited by J. Boxill. Oxford: Blackwell Publishing: 267–72.

MAGDALINSKI, T. and K. BROOKS. 2002. Bride of Frankenstein: Technology and the consumption of the female athlete. In *Sport Technology: History, Philosophy and Policy*, edited by A. Miah and S.B. Eassom. Amsterdam, Boston, MA, and London: Elsevier Science Ltd: 195–212.

MIAH, A. 2003. Be very afraid: Cyborg athletes, transhuman ideals and posthumanity. *Journal of Evolution and Technology* 13. Available at http://jetpress.org/volume13/miah/html, accessed October 2005.

———. 2004. *Genetically Modified Athletes: Biomedical Ethics, Gene Doping and Sport*. London and New York: Routledge.

MOI, T. 1999. *What is a Woman? And Other Essays*. Oxford; Oxford University Press.

MOLLER OKIN, S.M. 1979. *Women in Western Political Thought*. Princeton, NJ, and Guildford: Princeton University Press.

MUNTHE, C. 2000. Selected champions: Making winners in the age of genetic technology. In *Values in Sport: Elitism, Nationalism, Gender Equality and the Scientific Manufacture of Winners*, edited by T. Tännsjö and C. Tamburrini. London and New York: E & FN Spon: 217–31.

NORDQVIST, K. and A. ERIKSSON. 2004. Kvinna eller man ['Woman or man']. *Forskning & Framsteg* 1: 18–22.

ROWLAND, R. 1984. Reproductive technologies. The final solution to the woman question? In *Test-Tube Women. What Future for Motherhood?* edited by R. Arditti, R. Duelli Klein and S. Minden. London, Boston, MA, Melbourne and Henley: Pandora Press: 356–71.

RUBIN, G. 1975. The traffic in women: Notes on the 'political economy' of sex. In *Toward an Anthropology of Women*, edited by R. Rayna and R. Reiter. New York and London: Monthly Review Press: 157–210.

SANDELL, K. 2003. Att operera kroppen för att bli 'riktig' kvinna?! ['Reconstructing the body in order to become a 'real' woman?!'] In *Feministiska tolkningar av kosmetisk kirurgi* ['*Feminist interpretations of cosmetic surgery*'], In, Mer än bara kvinnor och män. Feministiska perspektiv på genus. ['More than just women and Men. Feminist perspectives on gender'], edited by D. Mulinari, K. Sandell and E. Schömer. Lund: Studentlitteratur: 189–213.

SHELLEY, M. 1959. *Frankenstein*. Stockholm: Christofers bokförlag (orig. pub. 1818).

SHERWIN, S. and M. SCHWARTZ. 2005. Resisting the emergence of Bio-Amazons. In *Genetic Technology and Sport – Ethical Questions*, edited by C. Tamburrini and T. Tännsjö. London and New York: Routledge: 199–204.

SHOGAN, D. 2002. Disciplinary technologies of sport performance. In *Sport Technology: History, Philosophy and Policy*, edited by A. Miah and S.B. Eassom. Amsterdam, Boston, MA, and London: Elsevier Science Ltd: 93 – 109.

SKIRSTAD, B. 2000. Gender verification in competitive sport: turning from research to action. In *Values in Sport: Elitism, Nationalism, Gender Equality and the Scientific Manufacture of Winners*, edited by T. Tännsjö and C. Tamburrini. London and New York: E & FN Spon: 116 – 22.

SÖDERBERG, H. 2004. Hårdare krav för transsexuella ['Stronger requirements for transsexuals']. *Svensk idrott* 6: 23.

TAMBURRINI, C. and T. TÄNNSJÖ. 2005. The genetic design of a new Amazon. In *Genetic Technology and Sport – Ethical Questions*, edited by C. Tamburrini and T. Tännsjö. London and New York: Routledge: 181 – 98.

TÄNNSJÖ, T. 2000. Against sexual discrimination in sports. In *Values in Sport: Elitism, Nationalism, Gender Equality and the Scientific Manufacture of Winners*, edited by T. Tännsjö and C. Tamburrini. London and New York: E & FN Spon: 101 – 15.

YOUNG, I.M. 1995. The exclusion of women in sport: Conceptual and existential dimensions. In *Philosophic Inquiry in Sport*, edited by W. Morgan and K. Meier. Champaign, IL: Human Kinetics: 262 – 6.

Index